VAN LIFE

First published in March 2019

British Library Cataloguing in Publication Data
A catalogue record for this book is available
from the British Library.

ISBN 978 1 78521 595 7

Library of Congress catalog card no. 2018953072

Published by Haynes Publishing,
Sparkford, Yeovil, Somerset BA22 7JJ, UK
Tel: 01963 440635
Int. tel: +44 1963 440635
Website: www.haynes.com

Haynes North America Inc.
861 Lawrence Drive, Newbury Park,
California 91320, USA

Interior design: Richard Parsons
Cover design: Mecob

Printed and bound in Malaysia

VAN LIFE

ALL YOU NEED TO KNOW IN ONE CONCISE MANUAL

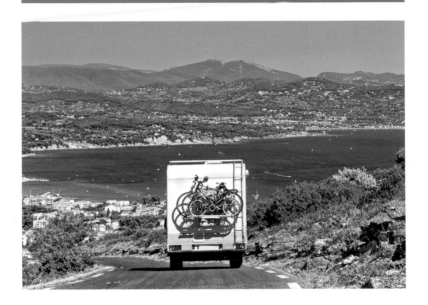

Haynes

Nigel Donnelly

Contents

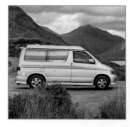 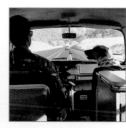 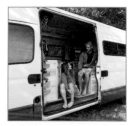

Van Life Inspiration

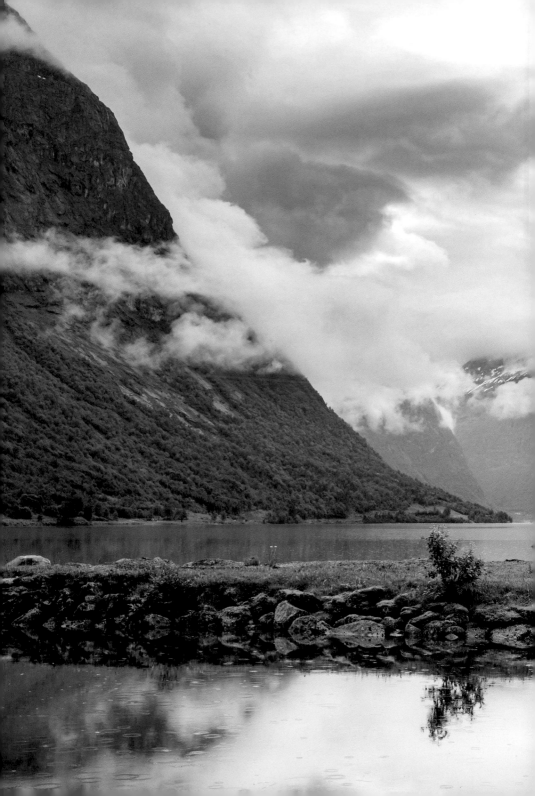

Introduction

Fly a thousand miles, you miss a million things along the way. What you passed over may be amazing, but all you've seen is clouds through a tiny window. Drive the same distance and it's completely different. You're not just travelling. You're exploring. Experiencing. Living. You'll find places and people that even the best guide books don't know about. Take what you need. Stop when you like. Go where you like. That is van life.

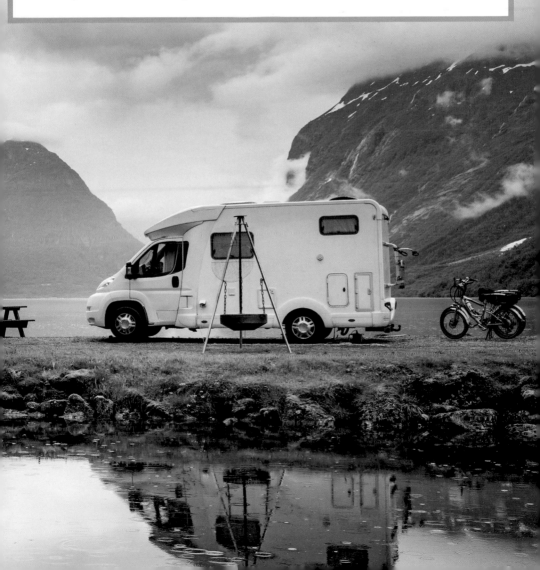

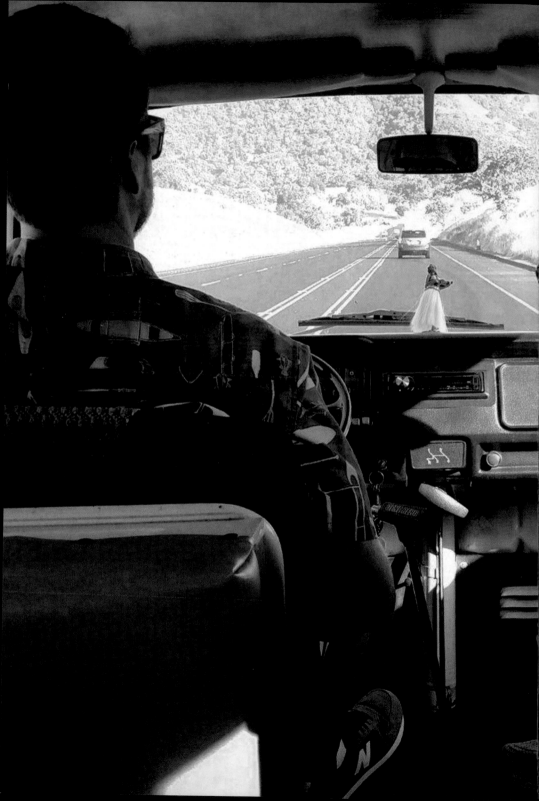

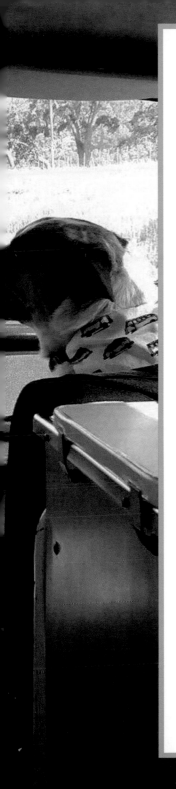

Chapter 1
Life on the road

'Vanlife is poetic in its simplicity that simultaneously encompasses and represents a lifestyle of living the way you choose to live, and going where you want when you want with limited "real world" responsibilities to hold you back.'

Foster Huntington, *New Yorker* magazine, April 2017

Van life stands for freedom

Van life. As a phrase, it is a modern one, but what it conjures up is as old as humanity. It is essentially a contemporary, catch-all term to encapsulate a life on the road. A way to live your own way, untethered by the fripperies of modern life.

The term was first coined by Foster Huntington, a designer in his late 20s who decided to move from his New York apartment into a 1987 Volkswagen Vanagon Syncro campervan. He decided to coin his own hashtag on a (then) relatively obscure social-media platform called Instagram.

As a graphic artist, Instagram was the ideal medium for Huntington. It is a mobile phone-based social network that supports simple camera uploads and brief captions. Searching for images is done with a hashtag. His caption for that initial image had modest ambitions, stating that #vanlife was a simple art project:

'I'm starting a photo project called #vanlife. it's a celebration of ships of the open road and the notion that, "home is where you park it." Check out van-life.net and submit a photo'.

People loved Foster's photos. And why wouldn't they? Broadly speaking, they were an idyllic collection of images of Foster, his van and his life without a fixed

⬇ Packing up your home, throwing the basics into a van and hitting the road is bang on trend.

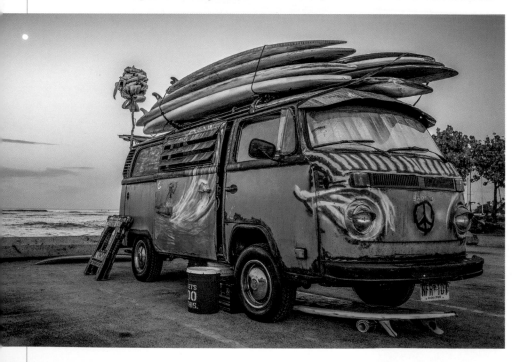

abode. This was no hobo life, however. Foster's van was cute, comfortable and framed by wonderful backdrops. What's more, unlike much of what appears on social media, it was not expensive, exclusive or unobtainable.

Others quickly started to adopt the tag. Many were van owners already, who sought to further illustrate the joy of a simple life on the road by posting their own photos. Many more were inspired by what they saw and started to visualise their own van life.

Instagram is literally a photographic memory repository and that means those images are still there today. You'll find it hard to dig them out though because the vanlife hashtag is now used on thousands of Instagram posts each day as people share their experiences, travails and views from the door of their vans. What started as a simple art project was now something of a credo for those seeking to declutter their lives. Van life had become a movement.

The modern nomads

Clearly, though, Huntington didn't invent the idea of living on the move. Someone who is constantly on the go rather than staying put is said to be a nomad, and it's a word often bandied around in the van life community. It's not a completely accurate description, but it's not bad.

The Oxford dictionary defines a nomad as: '... a member of a people that travels from place to place to find fresh pasture for its animals and has no permanent home'. In most cases, people classing themselves as nomads these days tend to do so for the pure pleasure of travel rather than because they are looking for more grass, but it's close.

The traditional nomadic communities came from all corners of the earth, all

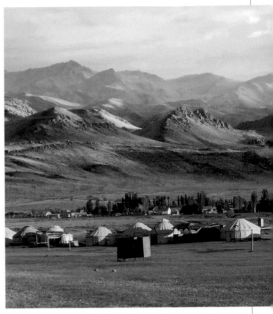

↑ These tents and vehicles in Kyrgyzstan represent a nomadic way of life that has barely altered for many generations.

faiths and all backgrounds. Some travelled to forage for food, others to seek pasture for their livestock or to find work. It was normally an ongoing arrangement, with groups moving with the seasons. There wasn't much choice involved if you didn't want to starve or freeze.

The question of whether the fact that someone has chosen to live for extended periods in a mobile home of some sort qualifies them as a 'nomad' depends on how flexible your definition is. It probably should. Although these modern nomads no longer rely on horses, canvas and wagons, many do travel with the seasons, fleeing colder climes in search of milder weather and new things.

Certainly, saying you are a nomad sounds more romantic than saying you live in a van.

Van life and politics

Living in vans isn't just about leisure. Many modern ideas of life aboard a van stem from the counterculture movement of the mid-1960s, when these slow-moving vehicles found themselves in the middle of a fast-changing political landscape.

Post-war babies had grown up watching television and listening to the radio. They were politically aware and felt it was their duty to vent their anger at what they saw. In the USA, a reaction against a political class hell-bent on overseas warmongering bound people together, but the movement also came to represent a push for social change on women's rights, drug culture, censorship and all manner of other wrongs all across the world.

People questioned many of the norms of modern American life, one of which was

⬇ Rajasthan, India, a cameleer stands in the Thar desert, with his dromedaries and two young helpers. In the background is their camp, which is moved as the nomads graze their cattle.

the idea of living in a house. The humble VW bus – a slow, stout, light commercial vehicle – became a symbol of the zeitgeist, alongside other old trucks, school buses and station wagons.

Everywhere groups of disaffected youth gathered, ramshackle collections of these weird buses seemed to congregate, often with tie-dyed throws and blankets spilling out of the load area, protest placards propped against the side and simple songs being composed within. Whereas the nomads of previous centuries travelled to find pasture and food, here the affluent American youth moved between protests to campaign for social justice.

These vans were frequently decorated – hand painted with symbols of peace and

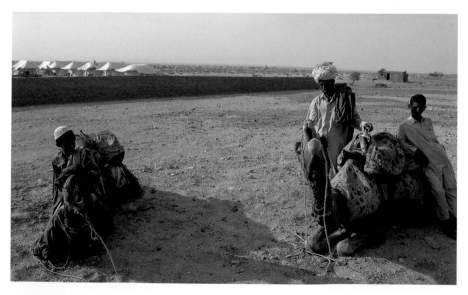

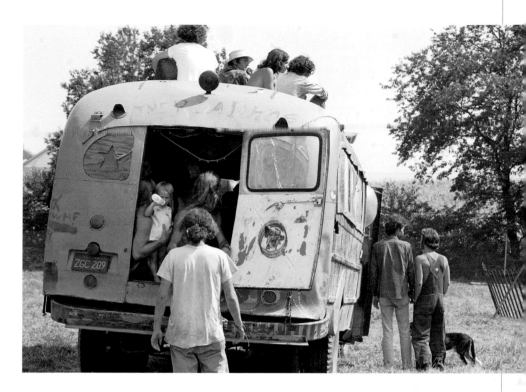

festooned with messages of love and tolerance, and the images of these vans at the centre of this cultural revolution cemented the status of the VW bus as the icon of the van life movement.

Protests pulled a lot of like-minded people into one place and they developed into transient communities. But you couldn't protest all the time, so music, drugs and sex dominated the downtime. Being politically active had never been such fun.

Having transport that was also an apartment made the job of being a hippy far more civilised. Being able to keep moving, however slowly, also made it easier to keep ahead of law enforcement agencies.

As time and society moved on, the fight for freedom provided by a van endured.

⬆ Hippies gather around their converted American school bus at the free Woodstock Music and Art Fair, August 1969. The festival took place on Max Yasgur's dairy farm, and about 450,000 people attended the three-day concert, which turned into chaos due to the crowds, heavy rains, and traffic jams. The vans, however, became rooted in the subculture of America's Summer of Love. (Getty)

Although the majority of hippies grew up, conformed, cut their hair and got jobs in finance departments, surfers still relied on their vans to let them overnight near the beach and be in the water whenever the tide was right. For bands struggling to get their music heard, a van was the way to move heavy gear and colleagues between venues. For others, a liveaboard vehicle simply allowed them to move on whenever the mood took them.

The rise of the RV

Of course, not everyone was taking on the establishment in the 1960s. Recreational vehicles in many forms were becoming available and affordable to the increasingly affluent middle classes. Travel trailers were built from the 1920s onwards, but it was in the post-war era that recreational vehicles (RVs), travel trailers and caravans began to appear in large volumes.

Initially, these were not fluffy travel vans to be used for heading away for the weekend. Wally Byam, the man behind the Airstream travel trailer, was adamant that his company built high-quality, robust trailers with an aircraft-style aluminium construction that could stand up to whatever travel adventures threw at them. He wanted to prove it, too, so he and wife Stella took vans to Europe in the early 1950s, covering many thousands of miles and visiting all the major cities.

Byam's company had started building trailers before World War II, with the plush Clipper arriving in 1936. However, problems with getting materials meant there was a break in production until 1948, but after that things really started to take off as the economy boomed.

The Wally Byam Caravanners Club International was an organisation that was set up for those who wanted to experience adventure in their travel trailers. High-profile trips were covered in the national newspapers, with 63 Airstreams setting off from El Paso, Texas to get to Nicaragua in Central America in 1951. Even today that is a tough ask. On unmade roads and with 1950s' technology, it was little short of miraculous that more than half of the trailers that set off completed the 2,000-mile (3,200km) adventure through Mexico, Guatemala and Honduras.

Yet that wasn't even the toughest undertaking. Byam led another group of owners on an incredible adventure, loading their trailers on to a ship in New York to start an overland expedition in Cape Town,

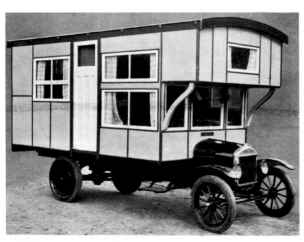

← The first motorhomes were elaborate, exclusive one-off coachbuilds for the well-heeled.

↗ In the 1920s, only the very wealthiest people owned a car, let alone have a caravan built to tow behind it.

→ The 1930s US-built Torpedo pre-dates official Airstream production but is a very close relative. (Airstream, Inc. Corporate Archives)

South Africa. The eventual destination was Cairo in Egypt – a destination that involved the vans travelling some 12,000 miles (19,300km) on roads that for long stretches were barely made or mapped. That 106 people spread across 36 outfits set out on this incredible journey suggests Airstream customers were intrepid and travel-focused – far from the stereotype of the modern caravanner. Byam's trip was planned to last three months, but it took more than seven. By way of context, efforts to repeat the adventure more recently were scuppered due to insurance difficulties and political upheaval. It is entirely possible that no caravan will complete such an adventure in the foreseeable future.

The European market burst into life at the same time, with a rash of producers popping up across Europe. Consumers were choosing to spend their leisure time in vans. This caused a corresponding rise in the number of campsites and campgrounds and offered the emerging middle classes a way to get closer to nature without slumming it in a tent.

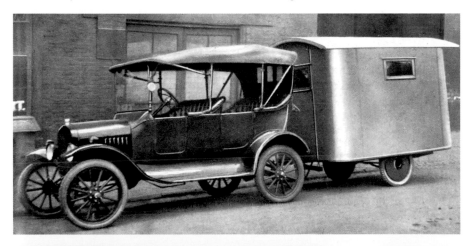

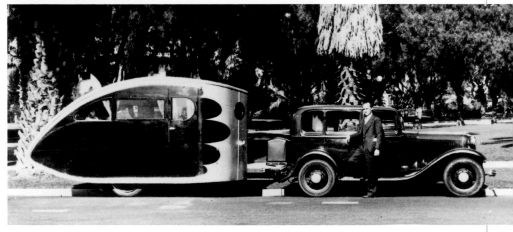

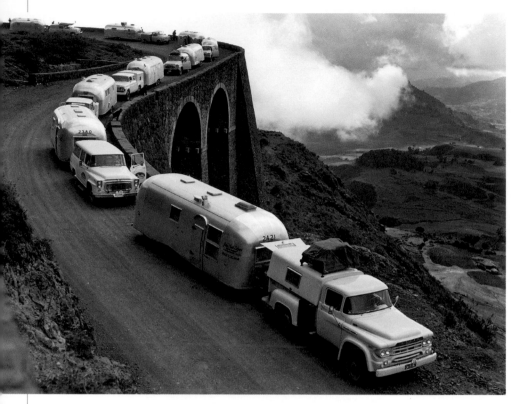

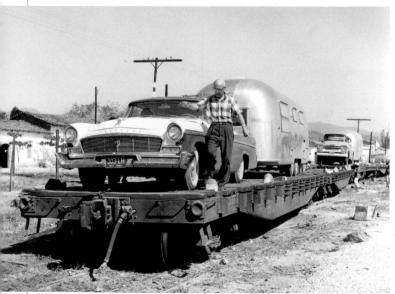

↑ Wally Byam went on epic trips to show the hardiness of his premium trailers. (Airstream, Inc. Corporate Archives)

← Trailers were moved by whatever means neccesary across the USA. (Airstream, Inc. Corporate Archives)

→ Caravans were a common sight on mid-1960s UK roads, thanks to Sprite who made touring affordable.

It was during this period that some of the big names that still exist appeared on the scene. In the USA, it was Winnebago and Airstream who pushed products into the market, while in Europe, Sprite, Hymer and Eriba all launched vehicles that brought van life to the masses.

The equivalent of Wally Byam in the UK was Sam Alper, a charismatic entrepreneur who saw great potential in the caravan market. Before World War II, much as in the USA, the market was small and the vans were very expensive. Alper's gift was that he could see the potential for a mass-market caravan that could be made more cheaply and would open up the touring market to anyone who had a car.

The first Sprite hit the market in 1949, but producing an affordable tourer meant people thought it was cheap and poor quality. Alper set out to prove otherwise. Whether word of Byam's run to Nicaragua had got through to Alper isn't known, but a year later, he hit upon the idea of an endurance test to prove how tough his cut-price Sprite actually was.

A three-man team hooked up a Sprite behind a Jaguar saloon and towed it 10,000 miles (16,000km) around the Mediterranean in 34 days. Despite mishaps caused by the terrible roads (and a runaway RAF Land Rover in Egypt), the fact that the Sprite completed the journey was widely reported in the press and the Sprite name was etched into the caravan-buying public's consciousness. Sprite went on to become a household name across the world by the end of the 1960s.

While the market has since weathered peaks and troughs in popularity as consumer fashions and tastes change, vans and trailers have always remained popular for those who want to live on their own terms. Whether running a plush motorhome to the Algarve or weekending on your doorstep in something more modest, spending time in a van for many means one thing: freedom.

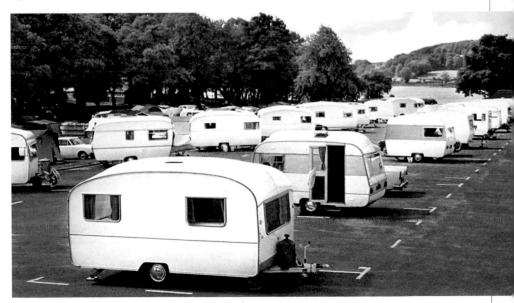

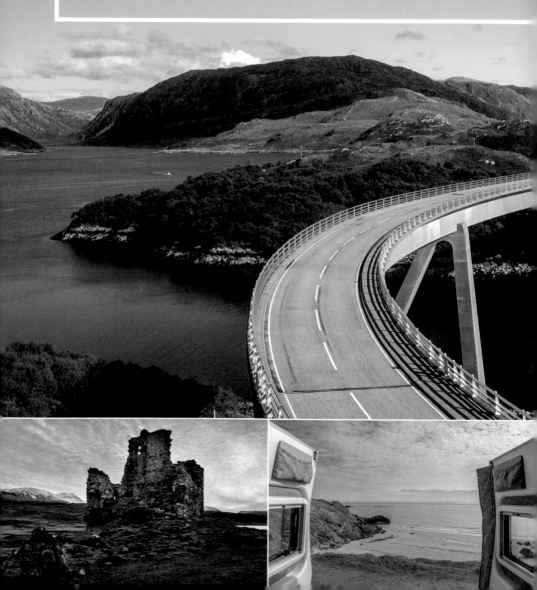

Van Life Inspiration
The Scottish North Coast

The north of Scotland is a glorious location for a van vacation. It's a long drive from many parts of the UK, but there are no sea crossings, and the reward is an otherworldly set of destinations, related to each other, yet completely unique in terms of tone. If you want to understand the appeal of vanlife, start here.

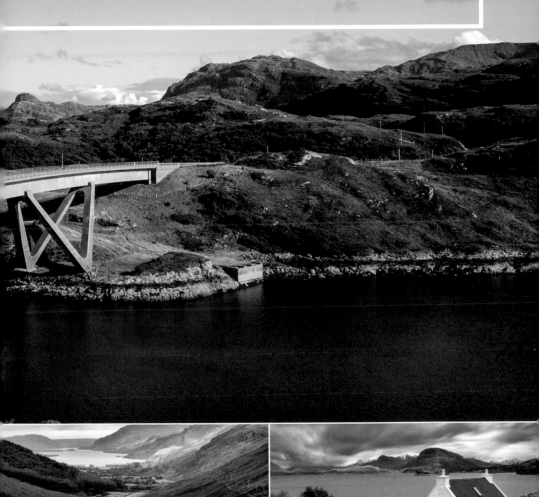

Digital nomad

While self-catering leisure travel remains a huge part of the market, since the mid-2000s, van life has been reinvented again. Much like the counterculture movement, this shift started with a lot of people thinking along the same lines, independently of each other, and all hitting on the same idea at the same time.

One of those people was the aforementioned Foster Huntington, but he wasn't alone – there were hundreds of young professionals working in tech companies who started eyeing up light commercial vehicles as potential homes.

During the noughties, the likes of Apple, Facebook, Google and many other major technology companies were (and are) based in San Francisco, and were busy hiring as many software engineers, product managers, digital designers and so on as they could find. This explosion in job opportunities brought lots of bright people from across the world to Silicon Valley to work but, being bright, they didn't want to waste their money on sky-high rents for poky apartments.

These were people employed for their ability to disrupt and to think differently. It was what they did. So, they looked for alternatives, and one of the simpler ones was to live in a van. After all, it was cheap, you could park near the office and if you had a laptop and mobile phone with a data contract, you could work from home. Living in a van also meant that your home could be parked wherever you wanted it to be. Want to take a tech job in Boston? Atlanta? Seattle? No problem. Gas up the van and hit the road. As van life became more popular, word began to spread.

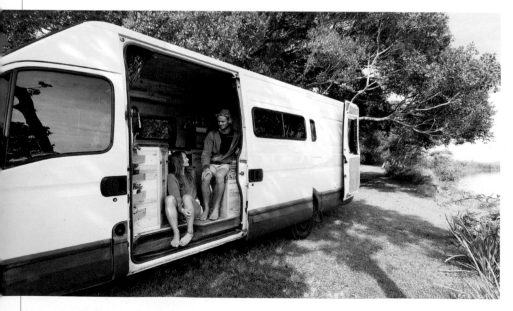

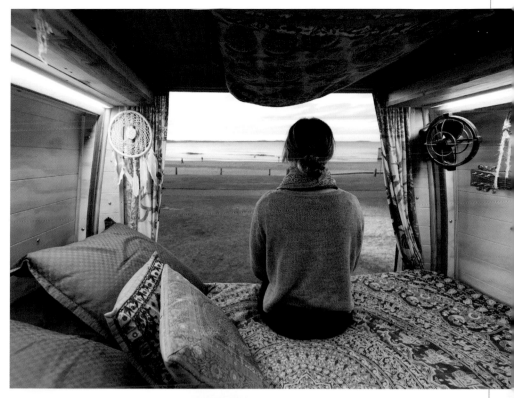

↑ A well-appointed van is the perfect answer to the problem of low wages in areas where property is pricey.

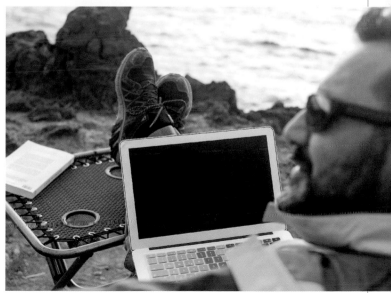

← Discrete vans with dark windows and few external clues, are as at home by the coast as at a city kerbside.

→ Many modern careers can be pursued any time, any place, so long as there is an adequate mobile phone signal available.

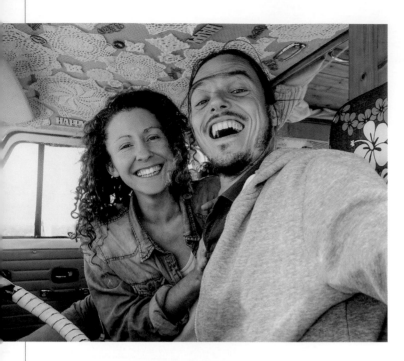

← Even the snuggest van is a nicer place to be than the plushest city centre office.

→ Not many traditional office blocks have the luxury of a view as good as this.

Information on how to find, purchase, convert and use one became popular online and a cultural phenomenon started to establish itself.

What was initially a practical way to save money while living in some of the most expensive cities in the USA started to meld with the idea of rejecting the mainstream way of living. Unlike the counterculture of the 60s, however, modern telecommunications meant that you could drop out and still have a job.

Typically, these van lifers were not looking for traditional RVs, which were too big and too conspicuous for stealth overnighting near busy city centres. Instead, the vans they opted for were regular work vans. From the outside, they attract scant attention, but inside, they are fitted out with a few comforts. Many have basic but entirely pragmatic furniture arrangements, including a bed, a small

working space, a basic kitchen and, in bigger ones, a washroom.

People who write software or do other digital roles don't need to be in the office to work. As long as they have a laptop, power and a connection to the internet, they are just as effective in the back of their van as they are in an office cubicle. Modern messaging tools such as Google Chat, Skype and Slack mean they can be in constant real-time contact with colleagues anywhere in the world. This makes them distinct for many leisure-only van lifers who use their vans when they aren't working, and with this new breed of van user came a new term: digital nomad.

These days, lots of companies outside the tech space are also embracing the idea of 'co-located teams' – essentially a way of saying that your colleagues are not all in one place sitting next to each other. While it is certainly not the case that everyone can

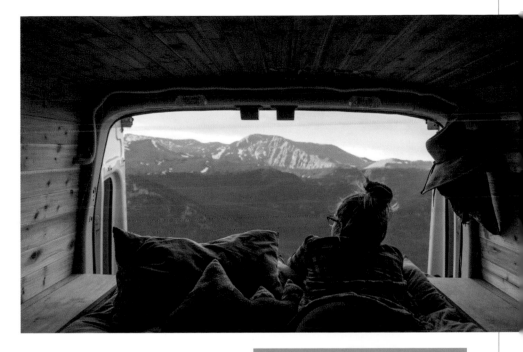

tell their boss they won't be in the office for a few months, employers are generally a lot more flexible than they were in the past, and that can be useful when it comes to maximising the time you get to spend in your van. It also enables you to break out of routines that involve you commuting at the busiest, and worst, times.

If you can work from home on a Friday, for example, there is no reason why you can't travel somewhere nice in your van on Thursday night to avoid the inevitable Friday-night traffic jams. Working from home can equally mean working from your van, provided that you can take your calls, wrestle with your spreadsheets or generally get on with what you need to do. Likewise, taking your calls from a van on a Monday means you avoid Sunday-night tailbacks and get an extra night enjoying wherever you have chosen to pitch up for the weekend.

Finding your van life

Definitions vary and people argue about whether 'van life' means actually living in a van all the time, chasing the waves and having no fixed dwelling, or whether it's sufficient to stuff yourself, your labrador and a Thermos into your van and head off to the Lake District for the weekend.

In truth, it doesn't much matter. Think of your van, whatever shape or size it is, as a place in which you can vacate everyday life for a while. Whether that 'while' is a day, weekend, month or until you stop is entirely up to you. We hope that through this book, we can introduce you to some of the key ideas and considerations that might put you on the road to whichever van life feels right for you.

Case study

Human	**Tom Dibb**
Vehicle	**'Pickle' the 1989 VW T25 Transporter**

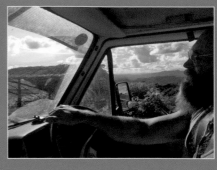

Tom Dibb is a singer-songwriter who found that plotting a path through the traditional routes of the music industry was getting him nowhere fast. If he was going to get nowhere fast, he may as well do it in his Volkswagen.

Tom decided that his best chance of getting his music heard was to take to the road. The idea of getting the gear and hitting the road is as old as the music industry itself, but Tom set his sights a little higher than a few pub gigs along the A1.

'The idea was to see if we could still get music to the masses the old-school way,' he explained, 'building a following by playing my music to the people who I met along the way.

So I hit on a plan to drive across 27 countries in 27 weeks with the target of getting to Melbourne, Australia.'

Tom took to the road in February 2016, with the support of sponsors and donations from a Kickstarter campaign to bolster his earnings from gigs along the way.

⬇ Tom Dibb's world tour bus was a more modest affair than many musicians enjoy!

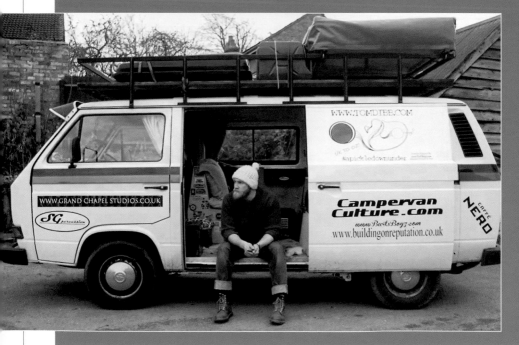

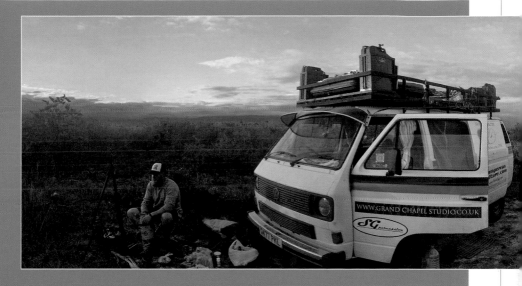

The route taken saw Tom and Pickle head through western Europe, down through the Balkans, across the Black Sea to Georgia and Azerbaijan, and across the Caspian Sea to Kazakhstan, Kyrgyzstan, China, Laos, Thailand and Malaysia before finally arriving in Australia in October.

The eventual mileage of more than 21,000 miles (34,000km) involved a total of 18 months on the road before Tom had Pickle shipped back to the UK in spring 2017.

Appreciably, there were a few unscripted adventures along the way, but any problems with the van or otherwise were sorted out and progress could continue. What's more, Tom enjoyed the whole experience and has fed this back into his music.

'It took so many years to put into place but it was more than worth it. I connected with people I would have otherwise never have met, walked among cultures I never knew existed, performed so many amazing shows and picked up plenty of attention as we went. There were a few hairy moments along the

↑ Tom and Pickle are now accomplished wild campers, and Tom is an expert at spotting suitable night stops en route to Australia.

way, but it all gave me so much material for my songs.'

After touching back down on UK soil in late April 2017 and being reunited with Pickle, Tom set to work putting his experiences into his music and the result is the album *Ground Up*, which was released in autumn 2017.

'This record is a culmination of everything I felt since sacking off my London day job years ago, planning A Pickle Down Under, and of course, all of my experiences on the road. I finally feel that I can share all I've seen with other people who are thinking about going on any kind of personal adventure. I hope people enjoy it; I hope it inspires people.'

Tom is a regular at various festivals and is a well-known face around the various VW summer festivals. The album *Ground Up* is available on iTunes and Google Play or direct from www.tomdibb.com.

Van life stars

Some vehicles are indelibly inked into the very fabric of what van life is about, and given what we have already said, this list of van life celebrities is dominated by vehicles from across the Atlantic, although not all the stars are from Hollywood.

Airstream

Airstream travel trailers are perhaps the only towed vehicle about which people with no interest in life on the road might say 'actually, that is pretty cool'. The first Airstream was the Clipper, in 1936, and elements of that original design can still be seen in the latest ones off the production line.

Sprite

The original Sprite models were launched in the 1950s, but the most enduring models are the ones built in the brand's heyday in the mid-1960s. Sold in huge numbers, they were a regular sight on caravan parks 30 years later. They remain highly prized in the vintage caravan scene and with a few basic updates are still very usable today.

Volkswagen T2 Westfalia

'Westies', as they are affectionately known, refer to VW 'Bay Window' models with interiors fitted by German coachbuilders Westfalia. There were several innovative layouts and many of these design norms established in the late 1960s remain in models sold today.

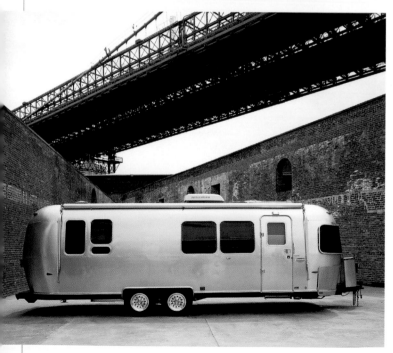

← A modern Airstream is the pinnacle of stylish, modern opulence.

→ The T2 Transporter is a ubiquitous sight, all over the world.

Definitions

Aire (or aire de service) – Designated stopover for motorhomes. These are prevalent throughout Europe, but are most typically associated with France, where there are thousands.

Caravan – Travel accommodation that you tow behind a car or truck.

Motorhome – Travel accommodation that you can get in and drive.

RV (Recreational Vehicle) – This typically refers to a large, US-built motorhome.

Wild camping – Spending the night in your van away from a designated parking area.

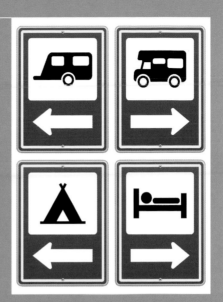

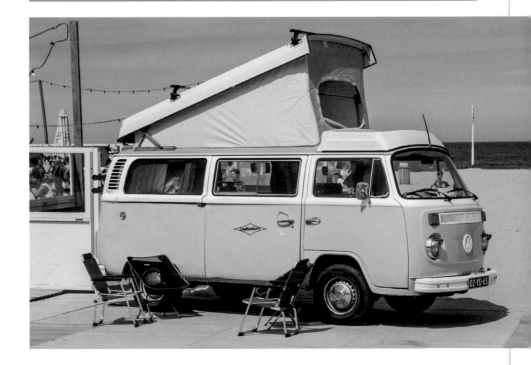

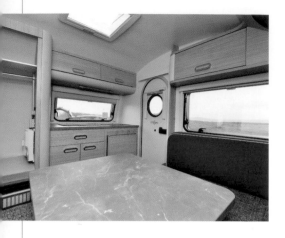

Eriba Touring

Eriba Touring models stand out from the crowd because they aren't built like regular caravans, having more in common with aircraft construction than anything else. As a result of the all-aluminium bodyshells, they last very well and the initial design was so successful that basic elements of the original remain in new models. They are also small enough to be towed by tiny cars.

T@B

By rights, T@Bs should not have been a success. They are small, meanly equipped and not very space-efficient. On the plus side, they look sensational, come in a variety of colours and are built to last. They are constructed in Germany but some models are also built under licence in the USA. They are great for weekends and short tours and are at the top end of the teardrop caravan market.

↑ The interior of the T@B is a masterpiece of modern minimalism.

→ The New Eriba Touring caravans still bear a remarkable resemblance to the 50-year old originals.

↓ The retro styling of the T@B has made it a modern classic. Wild colour schemes are available.

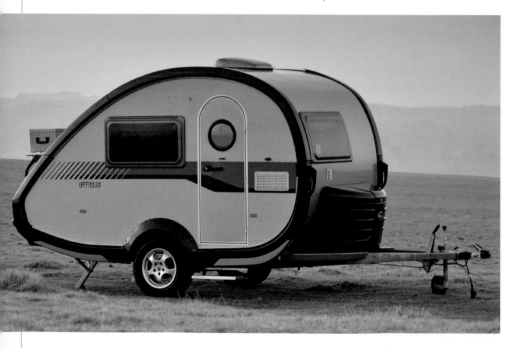

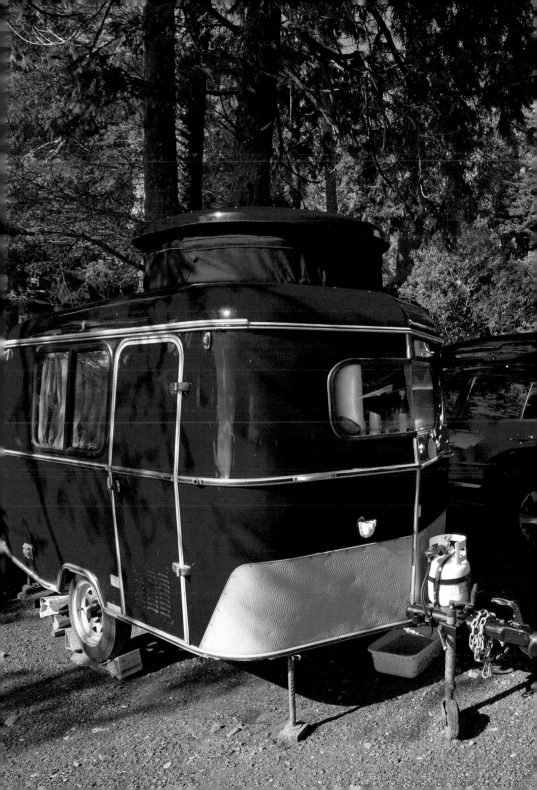

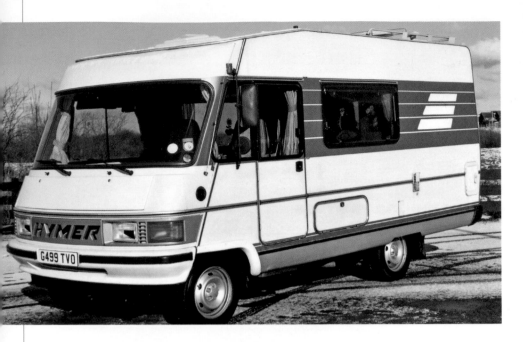

↑ Often credited as the original European integrated motorhome, the Hymermobile line-up remains the motorhome by which others are judged.

↓ The compact, rounded lines of the Auto-Sleeper one-piece GRP bodyshell were consigned to history in the early 2010s. It remains instantly identifiable.

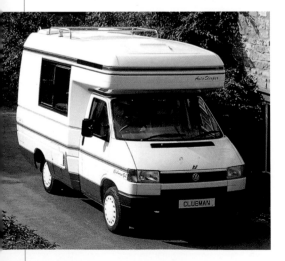

Hymermobil

The Hymermobil was the original integrated motorhome – meaning that the entire cab of the vehicle was integrated into the coachbuilt living area. The range was popular at its launch in 1971 and was eventually renamed the B-Klasse as Hymer's range of integrated models grew. The brown-and-gold ones made until 1987 were particularly distinctive, and built the reputation that Hymer retains for tough, practical integrated motorhomes.

Auto-Sleepers Clubman

The Clubman was a notable coachbuilt vehicle as it featured a unique two-tone, one-piece GRP bodyshell. A motorhome that couldn't leak was revolutionary. It was introduced in the early 1980s and lasted for around 20 years. The GRP shell made them heavy, but the strength it imparted meant you could have huge side windows, so they were very bright inside.

Skoolies

'Skoolies' are the yellow buses made famous by American films. They were made from the 1960s onwards and, in the USA at least, remain commonplace and simple to maintain. Alongside the Vee Dub bus, they are felt by many to represent a significant cultural touchpoint in the encyclopedia of van life.

Much like the original split-screen VW buses, while they used to be the cheap option, fashion has driven prices beyond the means of the budget traveller, meaning many conversions these days are expensive, designer affairs. Despite outward appearances, they aren't all the same, as they are built by dozens of companies and powered by many different engines. What they do have in common is that they have loads of windows so are bright inside, and there's a massive amount of space that can be filled with bunks, surfboards, motorcycles and anything else you might pick up along the way. Most are slow and fairly awkward to drive but they look great and last forever.

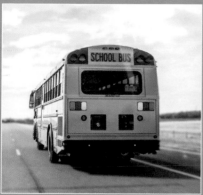

⬆ American school buses are widely available in the US and are a cult base vehicle among self-builders.

➡ The long chassis and wide-bodies mean a retired school bus offers a huge amount of space for blank-canvas conversions.

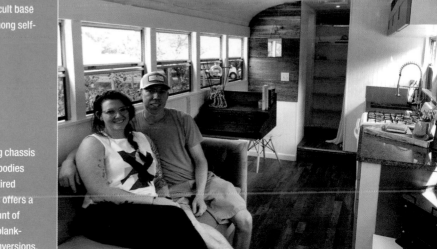

Van life in culture

The romance of the road trip is popular material for books and films, but pickings do get a bit slimmer when you are seeking inspiration for caravan and motorhome travel. Indeed, depictions of them in popular culture are broadly comic, although in truth, van life in all its forms is a rich source of comedy.

When it comes to campsites there are two *Carry On* films that prominently feature life outdoors. 1969's *Carry on Camping* is the best known, and covers a lot of the main stereotypes of campsite life, including a money-grubbing site owner, bad weather and so on. *Carry on Behind* from 1975 features caravans and similar scenarios, and was supported by the PR department of CI Caravans, who recognised a unique chance to gain exposure for their mid-70s tourer line-up on the big screen. *The Likely Lads* film from 1976 also features caravan holiday mishaps, including Bob and Terry crashing into the back of their own Sprite on a garage forecourt.

More contemporary laughs can be had with 2012's black comedy *Sightseers*, which involves a young couple's caravan break turning into a murderous rampage. It's funnier than it sounds. A celebrated episode of *Father Ted* from 1996 entitled 'Hell' details a weekend in a tiny ramshackle caravan and features a guest appearance by Graham Norton as a priest with a fondness for Irish dancing.

Motorhomes and campers also qualify for their fair share of laughs, and there are also some really good documentary travel films and shows featuring them that are worth watching.

Magic Trip (2011), for instance, documents a 1964 cross-country journey in a psychedelic school bus called 'Further', which is felt by some to herald the start of the counterculture era. The same type of bus also features in Tom Wolfe's 1968 book *The Electric Kool-Aid Acid Test*.

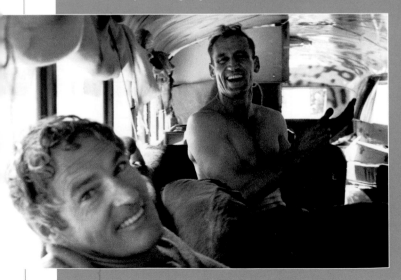

← The *Magic Trip* movie (2011) is felt by many to capture the zeitgeist of the counterculture better than any other.

➔ CI caravans played a starring role in the 1975 film *Carry on Behind*.

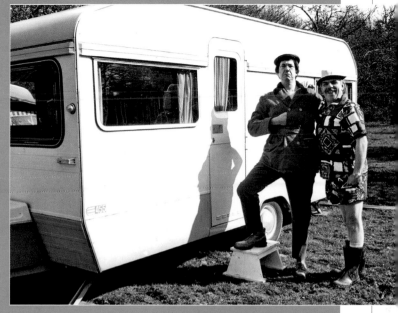

⬇ *Sightseers* has the caravan comedy horror genre pretty much to itself.

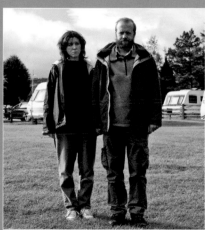

Of all the films, few capture the appeal and essence of van life as well as *The Leisure Seeker*. This 2018 film featuring Donald Sutherland and Helen Mirren tells the touching story of a couple who run away for a final adventure in their Winnebago Indian RV after Sutherland is diagnosed with Alzheimer's disease.

If you fancy something a little lighter and more knockabout, *RV* (2006) offers an undemanding watch and top-drawer silliness, centred around family RV adventures. *Meet the Fockers* (2004) also covers some of the lighter elements of RV life in some style.

For some more useful or inspirational watching, you can't go far wrong with YouTube videos from some of the very gifted, knowledgeable and experienced vloggers who make short films about their activities. We've included a list of some of the best at the end of the book.

More relatable to non-hippies is *Austin to Boston*, a 2014 documentary that tells the story of five Type 2 Volkswagens, each loaded with musicians who tour across the USA from the SXSW music festival to Boston and all their stops and breakdowns along the way.

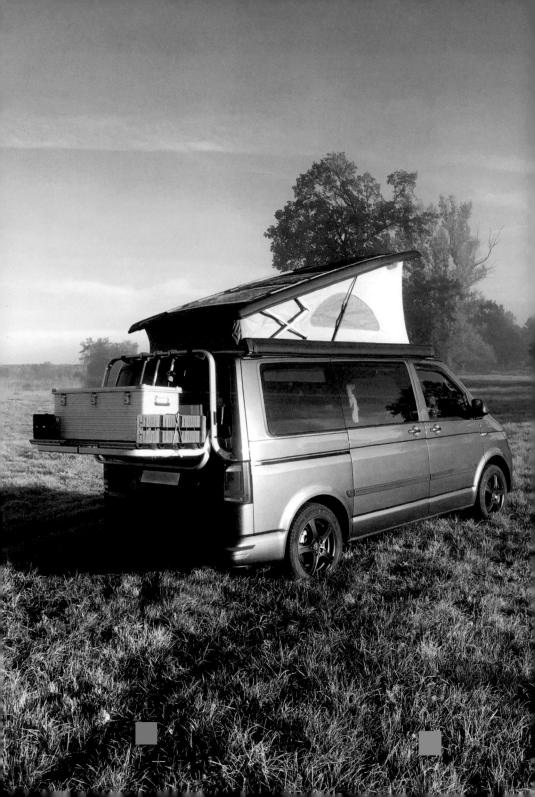

Chapter 2
You and your van

At the most simplistic level, there
are two basic types of van: caravans
and motorhomes. The difference
between the two is fairly obvious
once it has been explained – a caravan
doesn't have an engine, a motorhome
does. In order to go anywhere, a caravan
needs to be pulled by a tow vehicle.
A motorhome needs you to get in and
turn the key. There are different types of
caravan and different types of motorhome,
but we will worry about that later.

Caravan or motorhome?

Which is for you? You are the only one who can decide. If you don't know, read on. If you do, read on and let's understand fully the good and bad points of each.

You've probably already decided 'not a caravan' and it's fair to say they have something of an image problem. Unjustifiably. It's a purely British disease, too. Across Europe, caravans are just another means of having a holiday, whereas in Britain they are seen as a bit fusty and sad. This has not been helped by programmes such as *Top Gear*, which sought to cement the idea that a caravan was something to be ridiculed.

Despite the efforts of Clarkson and co, though, caravans remain very popular. If you are taking your first steps into the world of van ownership, it is worth spending some time thinking about caravans before dismissing them as a means of exploring. They have some advantages over a motorhome, so it makes sense to work out whether these are significant to you.

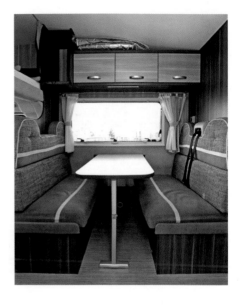

⬆ What is important to you? On-site comfort? Go-anywhere ability? Consider the decision carefully to ensure you get the van life you want.

Pros and cons of caravans versus motorhomes

	Caravan	Motorhome
Special driving licence	✗	✓
Easy to purchase	✓	✗
Lower running costs	✓	✗
Lower travel costs	✗	✓
Better interior comfort	✓	✗
Better to drive	✗	✓

Driving licence categories

Driving licence qualifications changed significantly in January 1997. If you passed your test prior to this, you are very fortunate. In terms of motorhomes and vans, you can drive anything up to a maximum authorised mass (MAM) of 7.5 tonnes without taking a further test. This gets you into the realms of small lorries, so any van is fine. In caravan terms, you can tow car-and-trailer combinations up to 8.25 tonnes. That's a lot. You have nothing to worry about.

If you passed your test after January 1997, however, everything is harder. A standard car licence restricts both B and C categories to a MAM of 3.5 tonnes.

We'll do the easy one first. Category C covers vans and a MAM of 3.5 tonnes allows you to drive a lot of heavy vans. In fact, most new motorhomes sold in the UK are in range, unless you want something massive. To drive vehicles with a MAM of up to 7.5 tonnes, though, you need to take

an LGV (large goods vehicle) driving test. This requires a medical.

For caravan and trailer towing, things are more restrictive. The car-and-caravan combined MAM is 3.5 tons or less, and the trailer cannot weigh more than the towing vehicle's kerb weight. For outfits with a combined MAM greater than 3.5 tonnes, you need to pass a category E test.

It's worth bearing in mind that licence categories are altered when licences are renewed on the holder's 70th birthday. Trailer restrictions are simple. Licence holders maintain their previous allowance to tow trailers, provided it is within the maximum towing weight of the car towing.

For van drivers, however, the right to drive vehicles heavier than 3.5 tons is removed unless they have requested otherwise. Drivers need to pass a D4 medical examination, which looks for a basic level of physical fitness, and pass the standard eyesight test.

← Flip over your driving licence to see which categories and weights of vehicles you are qualified to drive.

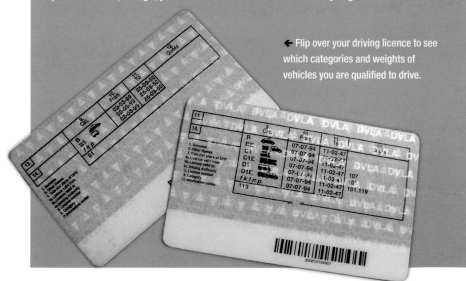

Money matters

Caravans are cheaper than motorhomes – both to buy and to maintain, although this is based on the assumption that you already have a car that can pull a caravan.

To put it in perspective, a new caravan with a fixed bed and pretty much everything you need for a holiday can be yours for less than £20,000. For the same money, you'll be looking at 20-year-old motorhomes. For £10,000, you'll have a choice of nice caravans in a range of sizes and specifications. If your budget is very tight, a caravan fits the bill better.

It's not just the purchase cost that makes a caravan a cheaper option, either. In terms of ongoing costs, there is no road tax, and essential servicing costs are around £150 per year. If your caravan is an older model, you don't even need seperate insurance for it – it'll be covered by the tow car's insurance when on the road, but you may want to consider getting additional insurance for theft. The choice is yours.

Things do even up a bit though if you are planning to spend longer periods away in your van. If your idea of a great travel adventure is to drive to somewhere beautiful, stay for a week and explore locally, then a caravan is a great bet. Almost universally, however, with a caravan, you must stay on a site.

Motorhomes therefore offer more freedom. On the Continent, motorhomes can use hundreds of overnight parking areas, which are cheap and often handsomely located within walking distance of town centres. Caravans are not permitted on these stopovers and have to park up at campsites, which are typically dearer and further from town.

Wild camping spots that permit caravans are harder to find, too, whereas

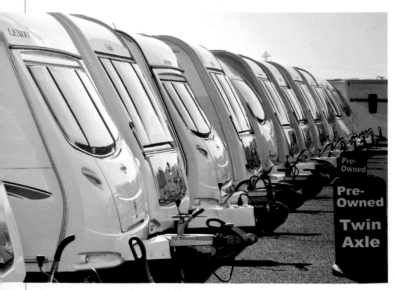

↗ American and Australian travel trailers offer vast interior space but need huge tow vehicles and open roads, and don't really make sense for European use.

← Your local caravan dealer will have a large stock of used vans to look at. It's a great way to get familiar with layout details, weights and pricing.

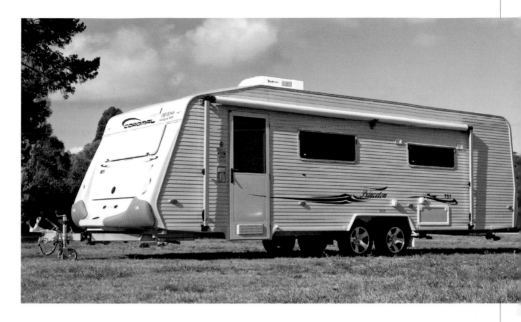

campers and motorhomers have far more options for low-cost, or even free, overnight spots off the beaten track. So, if a more freewheeling, ad hoc approach to overnight stops appeals, motorhomes are a better option.

Flexibility, then, is the most significant advantage of motorhomes; it's far easier to achieve constant onward travel, thus covering more distance, and you can be much more spontaneous and access far more areas – a motorhome can pretty much go anywhere a car can go, height restrictions permitting. That means stopping for a beach-side cuppa is a real prospect.

It's not all bad news for the caravan, though. Once you get to where you are going, you unhitch the caravan, put up the awning and are then free to go and explore with the car, while your temporary home waits for your return. If you are in a motorhome, every trip to town involves doing the washing up, putting everything

away and battening down the hatches. It involves effort. A caravan is the lazy option – in a good way. What's more, it's always easier to drive a car around town than it is a motorhome, and parking is of course also much simpler.

Another plus point for the caravan – one that is admittedly a little more contentious – is that regardless of how much you spend, a caravan is likely to be much more comfortable than a motorhome. The reason for this is that a motorhome has to have a cab at one end, meaning that a considerable portion of the interior space is taken up with a steering wheel, gear stick, single-glazed windscreen and cab doors. This is definitely a considerable compromise. Caravans, by contrast, have two useable square ends. Typically, one contains a spacious washroom and the other a comfortable lounge. A motorhome will only have one of those things, unless it's an enormous one, in which case this won't be an issue.

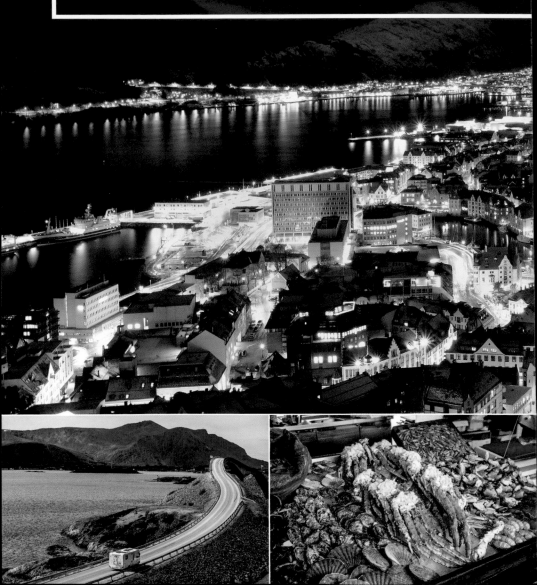

Van Life Inspiration
The Norwegian Fjords

Getting to the Fjords in a motorhome is a commitment, now there are no ferries east from UK ports to Scandinavia, but you will not enjoy landscapes like it anywhere else in the world. Solitude, politeness and vertigo-inducing landscapes are all in good supply. It is the very definition of getting away from it all.

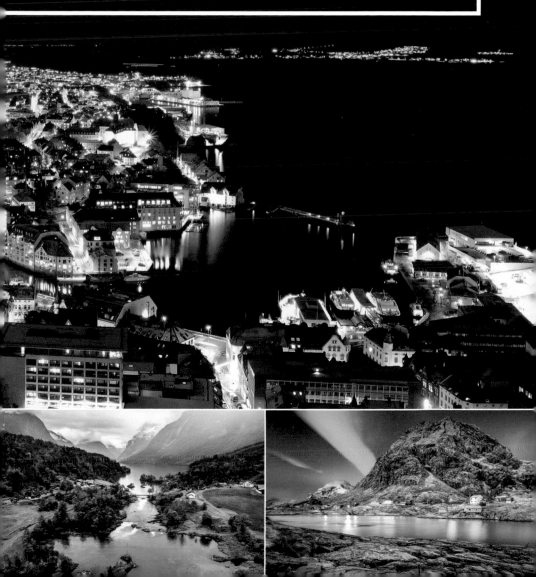

Outside the van

Unless you are very fortunate, you won't be able to spend all your time in your van and that means consideration needs to be given to where it will be kept when you are not living the dream. Storage is a serious issue.

For caravans and larger motorhomes, the matter is clear-cut: you either do or do not have space at home. If you do, then simply checking the dimensions of the available space will detemine what size van you can buy.

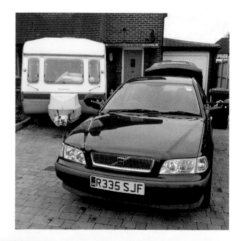

If you've not previously done so, it may be worth checking that there are no covenants on your home that prevent you from storing a van there. This restriction is not as uncommon as you'd think and is particularly prevalent on modern estates. It's obviously much better to know in advance, rather than to receive a nasty

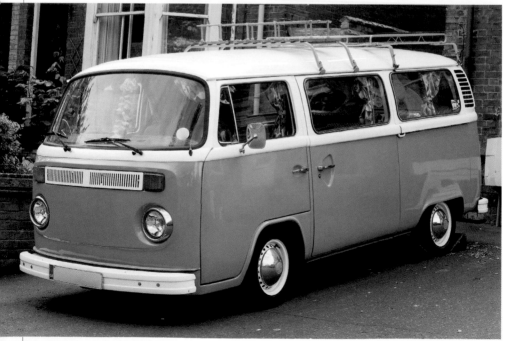

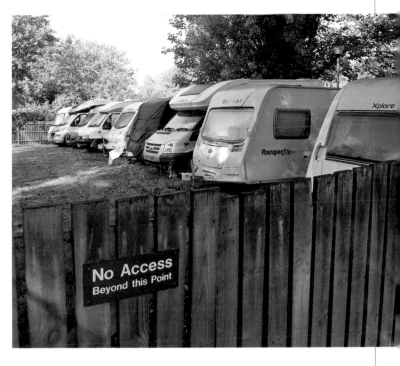

➜ Dedicated storage areas are the best option if you fancy a van but don't have the space to park it.

⬅ If you have the space at home, driveway storage is great value and convenient. Security and neighbour tantrums are the main downsides.

⬏ Smaller vans can be happily parked in the street and can even be used to replace your car. Newer tends to mean more reliability.

letter from a neighbour when you have a van on the drive, and then have to find somewhere else to store it.

A popular option is to invest in a dedicated storage solution. The best storage areas have security staff, CCTV, out-of-hours access and all manner of other protocols to stop criminals from getting their hands on your van. Alternatively, you could park your van at a campsite that offers secure storage. This has the advantage of putting your van in a location where you can easily have a quick weekend away as soon as the sun comes out. Often, however, they lack the flexibility in terms of out-of-hours access that a dedicated facility offers.

If you are considering a small motorhome to be your everyday transport, then getting something that is a size you are comfortable driving is the main consideration. Elevating-roof campers are popular choices in this instance, since they mean you can still access many multistorey car parks and they feel small on the road. Similarly, short-wheel-base models tend to be easier to live with day to day, particularly if you are parking on the street.

When you think you have cracked your storage conundrum, be sure to check that it satisfies your potential insurer. Many caravan and motorhome policies insist on a specialist storage provider if the van is being stored away from home. Taking advantage of a patch of land offered by a friendly local farmer or landowner may in theory be a great budget option, but it may not be good enough to validate your insurance. Finding this out after the vehicle has been stolen, or damaged, will be an unhappy experience.

Beyond the two-week break

Much of what has been talked about so far is geared around short- and medium-term stays in your van, but long-term liveaboard considerations are different again.

As the van is going to be replacing bricks and mortar, it is tempting to go large. That may be the right solution if you intend to stay rigged up on a site for weeks and months on end, but it makes sense to think in terms of the space you need, rather than simply the space you can get. Full-timers will often tell you that you should concentrate on finding a van that is as small as you are comfortable with, rather than as big as you can afford.

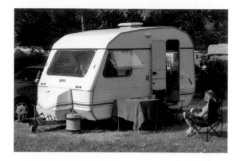

If your requirements are more specialist than those listed above, you've probably already got an idea of what you need. For overland camping or other trips off the beaten track, the emphasis shifts to factors such as good approach and departure angles, four-wheel drive, winches, the need for a storage garage if you need to take a motorbike, and so on.

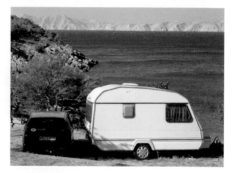

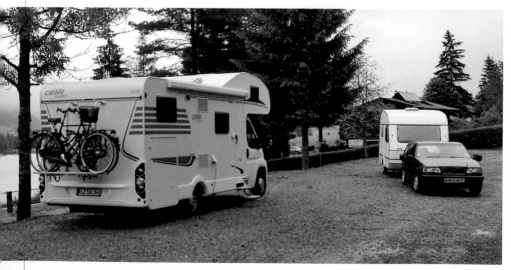

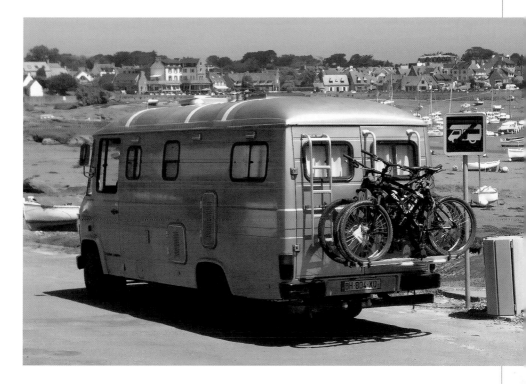

← Smaller car and caravan combinations are a low-cost way to hit the road. The Volvo and Sprite here cost £750 for the pair and toured around Europe.

↑ Motorhomes can generally explore a bit more widely and get closer to pretty places, but keep a look out for local byelaws prohibiting a stop.

Facing your fear of towing

A big objection a lot of people mention when choosing between a caravan and a motorhome is towing. The physical act of pulling a trailer is enough to freak out some drivers and if you recoil at the prospect of hitching up, then no amount of being told it is a good idea is going to change that. It is true to say, however, that towing a caravan is really not very difficult.

If you aren't sure, a great way to gain a bit of no-risk experience is to attend one of the big caravan shows that take place at the

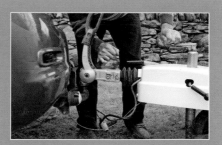

Birmingham NEC each spring and autumn. These offer free towing taster sessions, during which you'll get the chance to drag a caravan around a closed road circuit to see if it is for you. You might surprise yourself.

Case study

Humans   **Kate Lloyd and son Kyle**
Vehicle   **'Peanuts' a 1977 Auto-Sleeper, and a 2003 LDV Pilot**

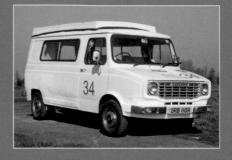

Like so many people with aspirations of enjoying a slice of van life, Kate Lloyd and her son Kyle were very keen, but distinctly underfunded, to go and pick up a motorhome from their local dealership.

'Mum and dad have always been keen motorcaravanners and I knew that having a van would mean that Kyle and I could have lots of breaks down to the coast to do a bit of surfing, go to music festivals and so on. I wanted a van, but didn't have a fortune to spend.

'We scoured the classifieds looking for something suitable. We didn't need much, but after sifting through a lot of stuff that was too far away, or just not very good, my dad found a likely candidate within an hour's drive of home. He knew what he was looking at and declared that this van was ideal for what we needed.'

The van Kate's dad recommended was a 1977 Leyland Sherpa with an Auto-Sleepers conversion. That means it was fitted out with a full furniture set and kitchen and the cab seats folded to make two single beds. It wasn't perfect, though. While 'Peanuts' was a proper little motorhome, age was definitely taking a toll on the compact camper and a pragmatic renovation started to take shape, with a view to making things a bit more reliable, usable and comfortable.

'We did a lot of work to tidy up the inside and make it more suitable for our needs. There were some pretty horrible bits of DIY to make safe, which dad attended to, all the while with Kyle inspecting the work and getting involved. It was great. It was up to the job, too, becoming the perfect beachside base for surfing and weekends away.'

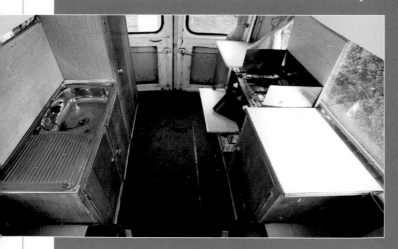

← Described as having a 'cosmetically challenged' interior but a new floor (fabricated from scratch) and a full MoT. Kate found the van a real retro-drive. The bus-sized steering wheel helped with the steering, however, and overdrive lifted the cruising speed.

Eventually, however, with the body starting to crumble and the mechanical parts having done 35 years of service, things were reaching the end of their lives. Given that much was right with the van, the obvious solution was to see if the best parts of Peanuts could be transplanted into something more modern to let Kate and Kyle continue their van-based adventures without massive expense.

Peanuts was thus reborn into an ex-Post Office 2003 LDV Pilot in 2013. These vans were a very familiar sight all over the country until a decade ago, so when they were retired from active service, sheer numbers meant prices were keen. They are also essentially the same vehicle as the Leyland Sherpa that the original Auto-Sleepers built into, so transferring parts was easier. It wasn't a straight swap, however, as Kate explains.

'We didn't bother transferring the roof as the new van had a different roof to the old one, which was taller anyway. And I'm not very tall! The new van had belted seats in the back, so we decided to keep two of them, and dad rigged up a bed that infills the gap between the front and rear seats. We fitted the original furniture we could fit in behind the seats, but rather than having a full gas hob, we swapped to disposable cartridge stoves. It means we can cook outside if we want to and we don't have gas pipes and cylinders to worry about. It's all I need.'

As time has passed, even the new version of Peanuts is started to show its age. With rust and a few mechanical maladies starting to take hold, Kate's thoughts are turning to 'what next?'

'I get so much use out of the van that I couldn't be without it. It's a big part of my social life, but with this van getting a bit tired, dad has his eye on another transplant,

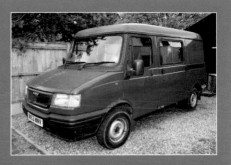

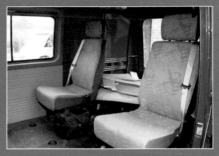

↑ Kate decided to look for an ex-Postman Pat crewbus. They were cheap, reliable, came with a full service history, rear travel seats, side windows and a semi-high-top. In 2013 she paid £1,100 for this 2003(53) LDV Pilot six-seat window bus with FSH, plenty of red elastic bands, and just 39,000 miles covered.

potentially into a bigger LDV Maxus. They are more modern, a bit nicer to drive and because it isn't a VW or Transit, you can pick them up for a sensible price. I'm not panicking just yet, though. We have just got a fresh MOT so there is at least a year before I need to raid the piggy bank!'

And as for Kyle? Well, he doesn't go away with his mum so much any more, but he's definitely caught the van life bug. 'He's built his own van now, and is just about to start on another. I am hoping he'll help with my next one, too!'

How much should you spend?

Van life is no different to anything else. It is easier if you have enough money. Regardless of how small your budget is, however, there is a way in. So long as you are satisfied with your purchase, you won't be excluded from the fun. We cover the buying and running costs of motorhomes and how to finance them in more detail in Chapter 3, but the following provides a rough guide to what different budgets allow.

Entry-level models

If you are buying at the lower end of the market, you need to be equipped with more practical and DIY nous to get the most out of your money. You don't need to be a mechanic or a cabinet maker (although it is handy) – you just need some basic DIY tools and techniques to get you going.

Older caravans in serviceable condition can be picked up for a few hundred pounds. Older ones are typically lighter than modern ones, which helps sidestep driving licence restrictions and means that you don't need a huge SUV to pull them. A normal family hatchback will happily tow a 1980s or early 90s caravan around without complaint. You will need a tow bar for your car if you don't have one, but for most models, there are options costing from just over £100 if you are prepared to fit it yourself. You could realistically be on the road with everything you need for around £1,000.

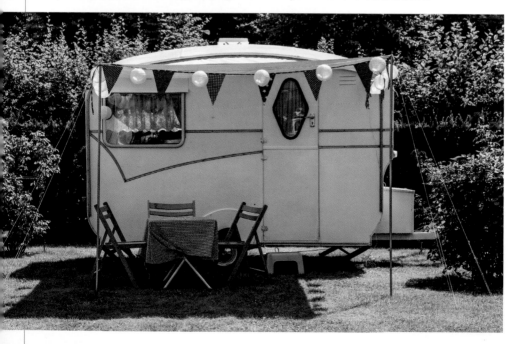

→ Keep an eye on noticeboards and shop windows when van shopping. It is amazing what comes up!

↙ Older models look great and can be tremendous value but your DIY skills will need to be on point.

↓ Self-building is a great way to ensure that a meagre budget is stretched as far as possible.

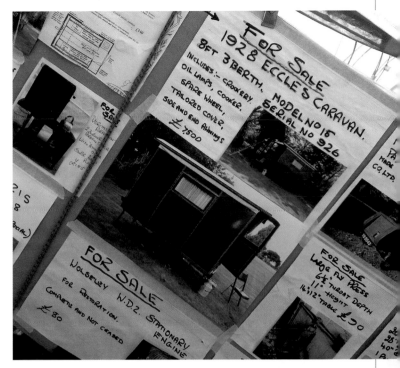

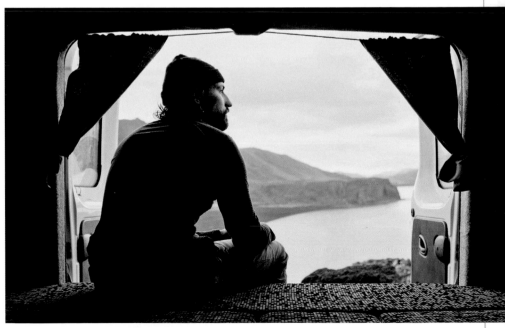

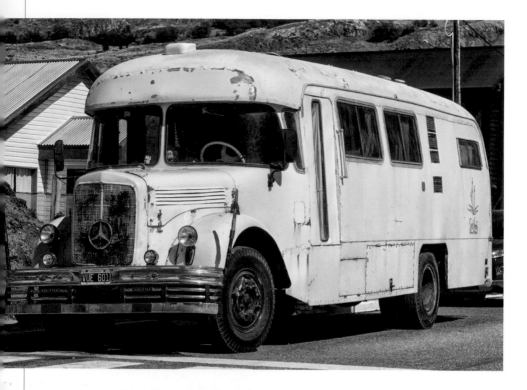

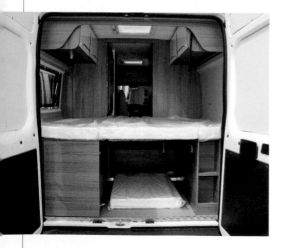

⬆ Feeling brave? A classic fixer-upper is an option for those who enjoy a (major) DIY challenge.

⬇ Bespoke modern comforts and convenience are tempting but come at a premium.

Starting points for panel vans are harder to judge. If you are building your own interior, you can certainly find your base vehicle for £1,000, but this is likely to be a vehicle that has had a hard life. If you are happy to take on some mechanical fixes and tidying up of bodywork, it's not a bad place to start.

Mid-range models

If you can stretch to £2,500, your options will be far better, as will the van. Look for older models with a lower mileage rather than newer ones that have had a hard life. Depending on your DIY ability and the sort of interior finish you are aiming for, you could well get a functional conversion in place for under £5,000 in total.

To stretch the budget further, many people seek out a caravan breaker from which to strip interior parts. Doing this can give your van's interior a more professional finish if it is done well, and often, items such as cookers, fridges and heaters can be sourced for hundreds less than their new equivalents.

With this sort of budget, you are just about in the realms of ready-converted campers (as well as fairly nice caravans). However, this is a tricky area of the market for motorhomes; it is a lot of money, but it is not a lot of money for a house or a commercial vehicle. You need to shop with care. Don't be disheartened, though – there are good deals out there.

Large motorhome dealers rarely have anything on the forecourt for under £10,000, so if you have less than this in the bank you will almost certainly be buying privately. As a general rule, interior problems are less serious than rust or heavy mechanical issues. Remember

where your DIY limitations lie, but if you have some skills and tools then you could get a great fixer-upper at a price you like. You will also find other people's DIY conversions that they are selling on may be on offer at this price.

Bigger budgets

Once you break into five figures, life is easy. Head to your nearest motorhome dealership and find something that you like.

Not only is this a quick and easy approach, but a more expensive, purpose-built motorhome or newer caravan will hold its value better and have greater potential when it comes to resale if you buy well and look after your van.

⬇ A caravan dealer site is a lovely place to shop for a modern van. You might even get a coffee if they think you are a serious buyer.

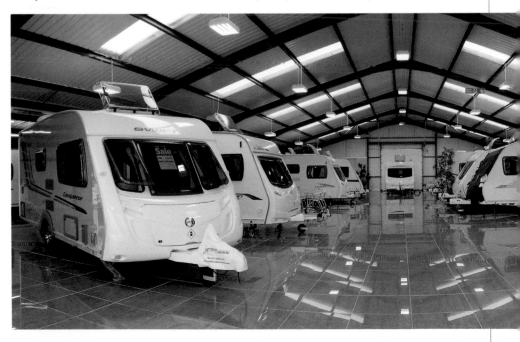

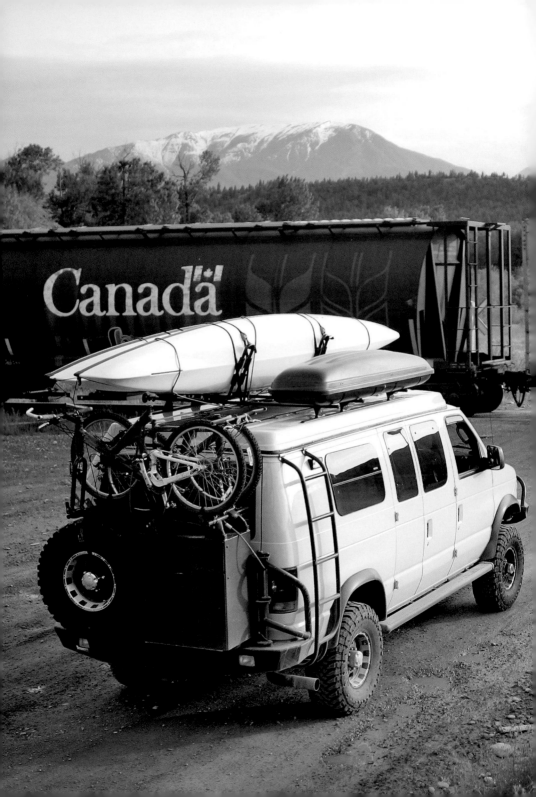

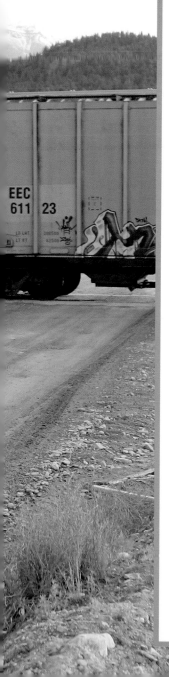

Chapter 3
Campervans and motorhomes

To most prospective van lifers, getting started means getting a van or possibly a truck – something that started out as a commercial vehicle and is now enjoying a second life as a mobile apartment. In these days of ebay, Gumtree and other online shop windows, it is incredibly easy to buy a van, but that is precisly the reason why it is so easy to get things wrong. With a little bit of planning, however, it is just as simple to purchase the right van as the wrong one, so you might as well do it right!

What is a motorhome?

We said earlier that a motorhome is distinct from a caravan because it has an engine – the accommodation is part of the vehicle, rather than being towed by a vehicle. That is a very broad definition, though, so it's time to categorise the different types to help you when out shopping.

Every motorhome on the market can be split into one of two basic types, but those types can get a little blurry. We'll do our best to explain.

Conversion

This is a vehicle that ostensibly looks like a van. They may have elevating roofs and most have additional windows and other adaptations, but essentially these look like close relatives of a standard panel van.

⬇ High-top conversions offer a great combination of on-road manageability and on-site space.

TYPES OF CONVERSION

Conversions come in a few different varieties. Vans that look too small to live in but have a simple camping set-up inside are referred to as campers or campervans. They often have pop-up roofs to give a little extra living room. They are easy to drive and park but most have no dedicated washroom facility, and if they don't have the lifting roof, you can't stand up in them. They can sneak under many height barriers, though, meaning you can access places that no other motorhome can.

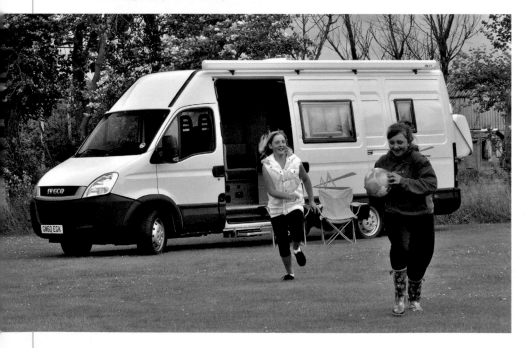

Conversion Case Study

The interior of Eileah Ohning's Freightliner Sprinter High Top van pictured on 15 July 2017 in Columbus, Ohio. A 31-year-old woman has turned her back on expensive rents and property prices – by living full time in a van. With an interior measuring just 13ft 2in long, 5ft 8in wide and 6ft 2in high, Eileah Ohnings home is her Freightliner Sprinter High Top van. The photographic producer from Columbus, Ohio, has lived in her compact four-wheel home since May 2017. Complete with a memory foam mattress, storage compartments, a desk and a camping stove, she even has plans to add in a shower, toilet and fridge. Eileah parks her van close enough to her workplace that she never needs to worry about the morning commute and showers at her local gym.

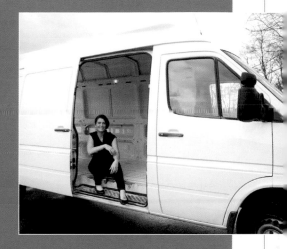

⬆ The Freightliner Sprinter is a close cousin of the European Mercedes Sprinter.

⬇ A combination of patience and talent, together with a reasonable budget, can yield incredible results, as Eileah's home-build interior shows.

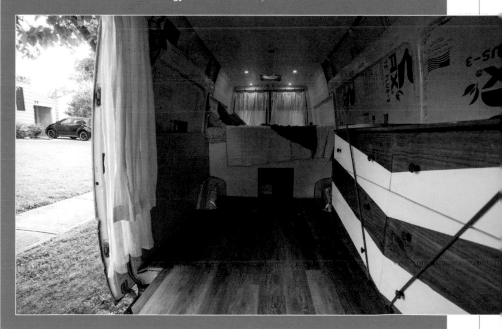

Van-conversion or high-roof variants have been a big growth area in the market in recent years. They look like a normal van, so aren't intimidating to drive, but have full standing headroom and all the kit you need to wild camp. This type of vehicle is the sort of thing tackled by the majority of self-builders, as most of the effort can be concentrated inside the van.

Coachbuilt

This refers to vehicles with bodies that are purpose built and mounted on a chassis. Some retain the cab of the original van, with a purpose-built body mounted behind, while others encompass the whole vehicle, including the cab in the bodyshell.

TYPES OF COACHBUILT

Vans with a purpose-built body have significant advantages once you are on site, the main one being the extra space on offer. Headroom is generally unrestricted, washrooms are larger and more comfortable, and the beds tend to be bigger, too. There are three basic types:

⬇ Pop-top campers are short on space but can go pretty much anywhere a car can.

- If there is a large bed above the driver and passenger seats, it is called an overcab motorhome. This is still a layout favoured by families, though they have fallen in popularity in recent years.
- If there is nothing, or maybe just a small storage area, over the driver, it is called a low-profile coachbuilt. They tend to look a little more handsome and may do a little more to the gallon.
- A further type of coachbuilt is the ones that don't have a separate cab, with the entire vehicle having a coachbuilt body. These are called A-class motorhomes, although they are popularly referred to as integrated motorhomes on the Continent. These are expensive.

American RVs tend to be categorised in parallel with these classifications, either as coachbuilt overcabs or A-class models, but they aren't directly comparable. Loaded to the gunwales with kit, they are a leftfield choice, but depending on your usage, they may be perfect. We'll discuss them later on.

⬇ Overcab coachbuilts have a large bed area mounted above the driver's seat.

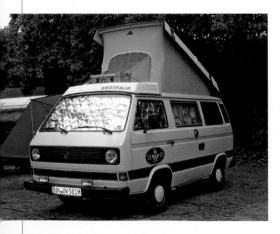

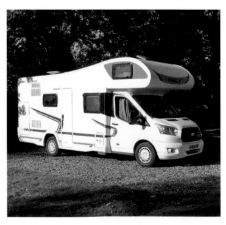

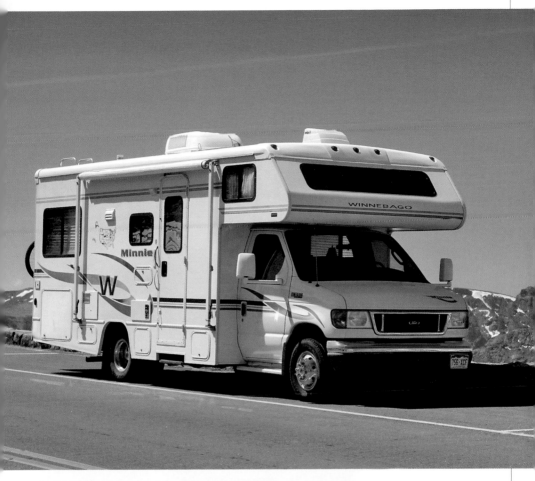

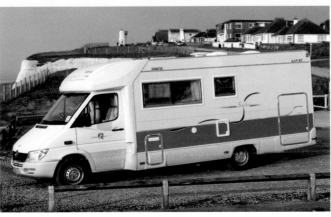

⬆ Smaller American RVs such as this 'Minnie Winnie' are good value but are typically thirsty.

⬅ Low-profile coachbuilts are more streamlined, and are typically sold as luxury two-berth models.

Case study

Humans	**Donna and Phil Garner**
Vehicle	**'Monty' the 1999 Ford Herald Squire 300e**

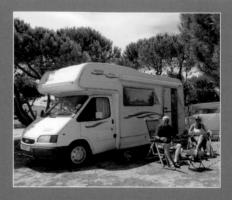

Donna and Phil Garner have progressed to a life on wheels after first sampling life on water. The motivations, however, are similar: the idea of having life a little more on your own terms.

'It was back in 2003,' Donna explains, 'Phil and I sold up and moved on to our classic wooden yacht, along with two of my three teenagers. We'd had enough of the hamster wheel of life, working just to pay a mortgage and household bills, and were in search of a more adventurous way of life.'

'This was great for a while, but fast forward to 2009 and the children had left to live their own lives, leaving Phil and myself to handle a yacht that was too big for our needs. That was when we started thinking about what we wanted to do next. We decided to head to dry land to explore in a different way.'

'We swapped to a 1999 Ford Herald Squire 300e, which we still have. I guess you'd call us "nearly full-timers" now, as we intersperse

↓ Full-timing does not necessarily mean you need a huge rig. Donna and Phil's compact coachbuilt has been their permanent home for nearly a decade.

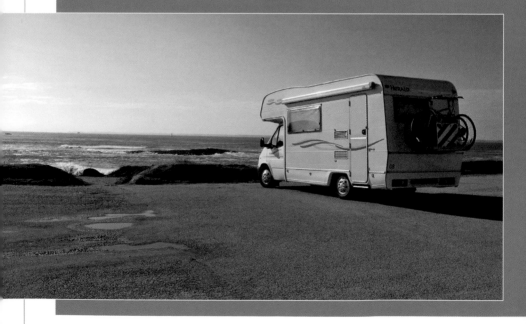

living in "Monty" the motorhome with spells of house-sitting. It stops us from going stir crazy or divorcing!'

Donna and Phil's favoured locations are popular spots with UK explorers, who typically head in search of fine food and weather on the Continent.

'We spend much of our time touring in Europe, especially France and Spain. There are so many aires to choose from in France that touring there is a doddle. Southern Spain is our go-to destination for most winters, for the relatively warm, dry weather, but northern Spain is beautiful, too. The northern mountain range called the Picos de Europa really takes some beating, especially in the summer months, when you can wander along in jeans and a T-shirt, looking at the breathtaking snow-capped mountain views.'

Donna is clear, however, that such a freewheeling life can't be easy all the time. 'It's not all an easy ride', she explains. 'Saying goodbye to family and friends is tough, especially now we have grandchildren. We also tend to have casual friends all over Europe, rather than a close-knit circle of friends.'

The Garners' Herald Squire 300e was a relatively posh van when new, but being based on a tough Ford Transit means it is easy to keep it healthy, although you can't predict everything.

'Dealing with disasters on the road can be difficult and is usually costly, too! We've sometimes had to rent accommodation for a while, or stay in hotels for a couple of nights, either because one of us is ill or has had surgery, or because Monty is off the road. When your home is in the garage for repairs, you have to find an alternative; keeping funds in reserve for this is imperative and one of the

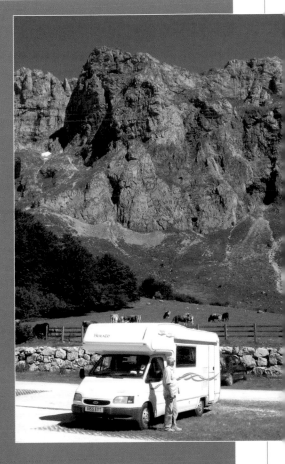

↑ The Ford Transit which the Garner's van is built on is tough, but simple to fix when it does need attention. Perfect for long-term touring.

main bits of advice I would give to anyone considering long-term touring.'

Talking through the ups and downs of things, though, Donna is positive that life in Monty suits them perfectly. 'There are downsides, of course, but living in the van really suits us. We still love our touring lifestyle and intend to continue living in this way for the foreseeable future.'

Choosing a motorhome

Working out which type of motorhome will suit you best depends on dozens of variables, such as driving licence requirements, storage and so on – as already discussed. Although these do need to be considered carefully, don't sweat over it too much; any motorhome will at the most simple level do what you need it to: give you somewhere to sleep and prepare a basic meal.

In fact, a regular builders' van with some insulation, an inflatable mattress and a camping stove to use outside is all you really *need*. It's just that some motorhomes will suit you better than others.

Campervans are fine, but typically they have little or no washroom provision. If you want to have a bit of self-sufficiency, you need a van with a washroom. For longer trips of more than just a couple of days, campervans can start to feel a little claustrophobic. In these circumstances, a high-roof van conversion is the next basic step up. These tend to be a little longer and a lot taller than campervans, as the name suggests; typically, you get full standing headroom, which really helps you avoid backache. Smaller vans with elevating roofs are another option, but those have you stooping at either end, and the routine of raising and lowering starts to lose its allure when you have to do it every time you move.

Another benefit of the high-roof van is that it is likely to have some sort of washroom. It will be pretty basic, with a

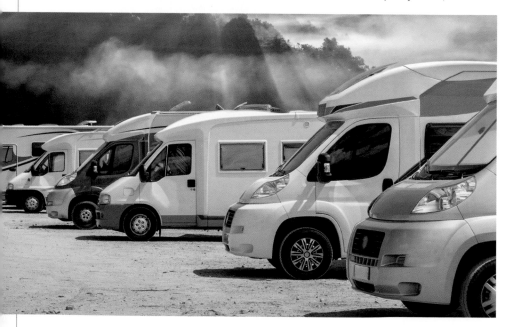

The economics of the motorhome market

Ideally, everyone would have a new motorhome. The latest ones come with loads of kit, are good to drive, reliable, economical and some of them even look quite nice. There is nothing not to like. Apart from the cost, which is the main reason why not everyone has one.

Making sense of the motorhome market requires you to open your mind a bit. The first thing to get out of your head is that a motorhome is like a car. It is not. A motorhome seems very expensive for a car, and that is because it is. However, it is very cheap when compared to a house, and it has a lot more in common with one of those than it does a car. What's more, a motorhome depreciates in value slowly, and with the appropriate level of care and investment will carry on doing the job it was designed to do. Ostensibly, that job is to keep you warm, dry, fed and watered, like a house. This explains why you can get finance packages on motorhomes that last for ten years and are much more akin to mortgages than car loans.

Such finance is also made possible by the resistance of motorhomes to the legendary depreciation that cars suffer from. Motorhomes just don't lose value in the same way. A posh car may retain 46 per cent of its value after three years; a new motorhome retains around 70 per cent of its value after three years.

Why does this matter? Well, if you spend a lot of money on acquiring a van, there is an excellent chance you will get a lump sum back later on. Think of it as money invested rather than money spent.

modest toilet and probably a poky shower, but its presence does open up overnight locations that have no facilities, such as certified camping club sites and overnight aire motorhome stops on the Continent.

Coachbuilt motorhomes are the next level, and offer much more space, which means better washrooms, kitchens and lounges when compared with those of a high-roof van.

For comfort, A-class motorhomes offer the fewest compromises on site but are the most cumbersome on the road. This is offset by the fact that they have no narrow cab area at the front, which means that the lounges are better and they have a large, wide, drop-down bed over the cab. For long-term or full-time touring, they are the best there is.

⬇ There is a huge variety of motorhome types to pick between. Head to a show to weigh up the range of options.

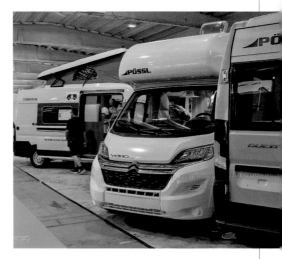

Money matters

The simplest route to life on the road is to visit a dealership, have a poke around the tin on display in the forecourt and pick something. There is nothing at all wrong with this approach, and, frankly, anyone who says there is, is probably just jealous.

We say 'jealous' because this approach requires money. Or at least a reasonable credit score. It's very hard to talk specific prices, but for a new coachbuilt motorhome you will be looking at something around the £40,000 mark to get started. If you are considering second-hand models at the same dealership, prices tend to start somewhere just north of £20,000.

If this is feeling a little out of reach, all is not lost. Bigger dealerships don't tend to stock older, more affordable metal, but there are vans out there for more sensible money, contrary to what a dealer may lead you to believe. Heading to smaller

dealerships and looking around privately will bring a lot more affordable stock into play, but correspondingly, you'll need to be a little more careful; not particularly because people are trying to catch you out or turn you over, but because older vehicles, like older people, are more likely to be carrying a few war wounds.

Buying an older motorhome does not necessarily mean buying a fading wreck, but you do need to be realistic about the ongoing costs of keeping an older vehicle in good health.

That said, a good used motorhome is a smart purchase: it means that the previous owner takes the biggest depreciative hit

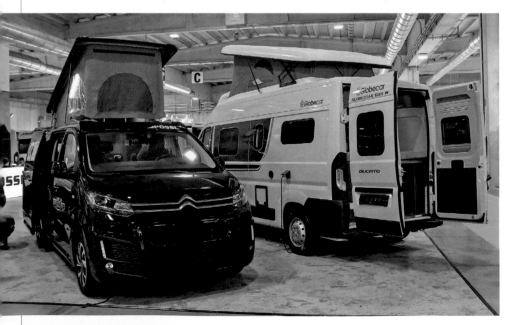

and at the same time allows you to reap the reward of their investment. After all, these vehicles are designed to give good service up to six-figure mileages, yet the majority of motorhomes cover very low distances, meaning mechanical wear is minimal. Spending money where required on maintenance is vital, though, even if it seems to be running well; skimp on it, and a frustrating time could await you.

We mentioned that thinking of a motorhome as a house rather than a car is useful, and this is especially true when buying an older, used one. The idea of buying a pre-owned property does not repel people, so why do some shy away from buying a second-hand motorhome?

Older houses often require a bigger spend when it comes to maintenance and improvements, but they don't become undesirable simply due to their age, and the same should broadly apply to motorhomes.

Car buyers are swayed by fashion, finance and how the car will fit into their lives, with considerations such as manoeuvrability and space for trips to the shops as well as running costs at the forefront of the thinking. A motorhome, on the other hand, has a very narrow specialism, much like a house: you need to be able to spend time in it when on holiday. Enjoying your break has a lot more to do with the weather, where you go and who you go with. There is no reason why a well-maintained older van cannot provide the same quality of holiday as one straight from the factory.

The key to staying happy with a cheaper motorhome is managing expenditure. Certain costs are predictable and can be budgeted for accordingly. For example, insurance and road tax need to be considered for any motorhome, as does the cost of filling the fuel tank. A good-quality breakdown policy is a must, too.

← Buying new or nearly new should give you some reassurance over its reliability, and the ability to travel long distances in comfort.

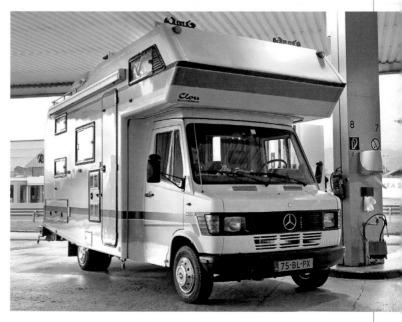

→ Older vehicles may cost less up front, but running costs rack up more quickly and journeys take longer. Find the compromise that suits you.

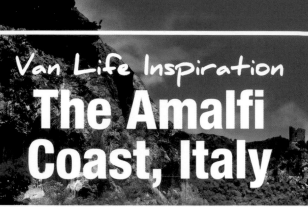

Van Life Inspiration
The Amalfi Coast, Italy

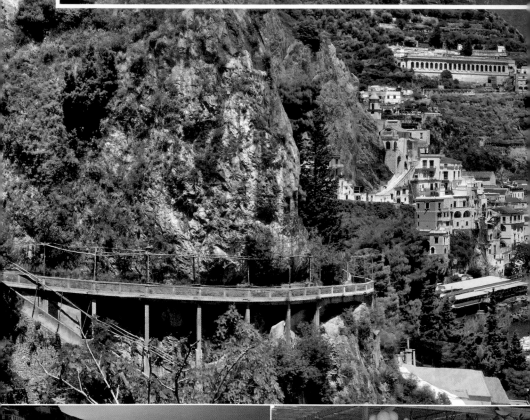

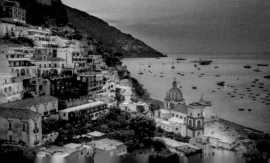

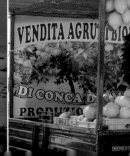

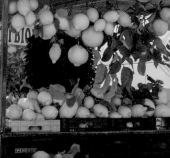

Large motorhomes are comfortable but there are disadvantages. The Amalfi Coast road is one. Big vans are banned from the coast road but smaller campers can savour the cliff-top trail. If you are oversized, simply park up in the campsites and use the cheap, frequent buses to get closer to the Limoncello.

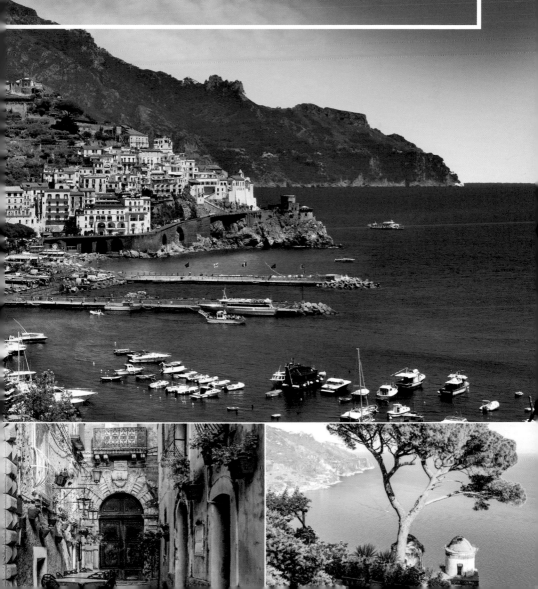

Self-building

If you really want to stretch your budget to the absolute limit and fancy a project, there is a special place at the van life table for those who build their own rolling homes.

Let's get the downsides out of the way early on: it is a lot of work, there are more rules than you might think, and it's still not that cheap – certainly cheaper than buying something off-the-peg, but depending on how you value your time, it could prove fairly costly.

Enough of that boring stuff, though. The pluses are obvious and many: if you are building your own van from scratch, you'll have something that does everything

⬇ You don't need to be a skilled carpenter to build a basic but comfortable, practical and desirable camping interior.

you want it to and nothing you aren't bothered about. If you need a van with storage for a motorcycle, a fixed single bed and a 44-gallon (200-litre) water tank, no problem – but you won't find that on the forecourt of your local dealership.

In the opening chapter we discussed the rise of the digital nomad and this group in particular has taken great pride in building their own vans. Many have done it with a focus on pragmatism, going for readily available materials and eschewing a lot of traditional norms of mainstream motorhome construction. The choice of base vehicle is different, too. By far the

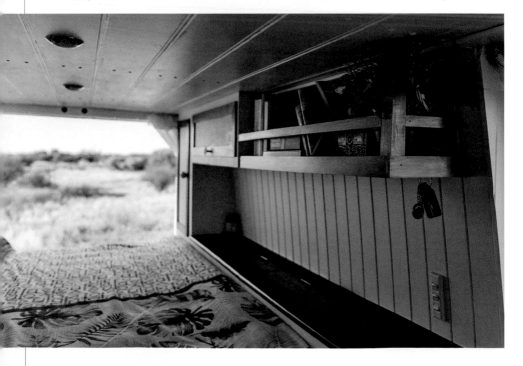

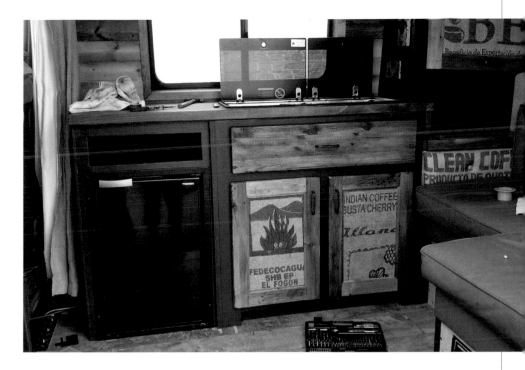

most popular base vehicle for self-builders in the USA and Europe is the Mercedes Sprinter – a model that's more or less an also-ran among mainstream builders.

The reasons for this vehicle's popularity are varied. Long-wheel base versions are vast and they have been around for long enough to mean that there is one for every budget. They are reasonably tough and pretty good to drive, although they do have a fairly formidable reputation for rust.

Layouts are diverse, but the common consensus is that the Sprinter is too narrow to allow for a bed that runs across the van, so most run front to back. Some are permanent, with huge storage spaces underneath, while others feature a long sofa that pulls into a bed at night. High-roof Sprinters have around 6.5ft (2m) of headroom inside before conversion, so only the tallest digital

⬆ If you like it, use it! David Howells used coffee sacks, plywood and leather to craft a stylish cabin.

⬇ The key to good outcomes is maximising space. David's van sofa converts into a bed base at night.

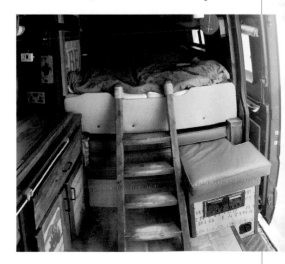

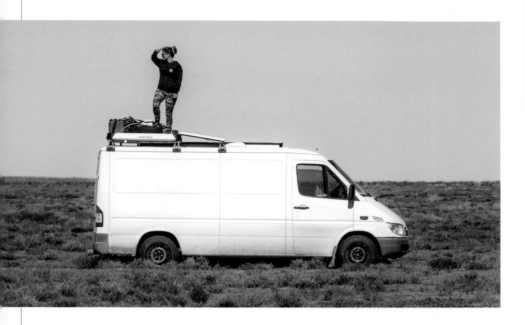

nomads have to worry about their head brushing the ceiling.

What makes a DIY conversion more appealing than ever is the amount of information available for those planning a project. A quick search on YouTube brings up hundreds of videos showing conversion work done by some determined and talented amateurs. Equally, there are some complete horror shows too, but they are useful in their own way as they demonstrate approaches that you might not want to follow.

It's not just YouTube, either. Instagram is full of inspiring build stories and there are dozens of Facebook groups detailing the work required to turn a humble delivery van into a fully equipped home on wheels. There are many great Facebook groups for self-builders, and the excellent forum of the Self Build Motor Caravanners Club (SBMCC) will become a second home should you break out the tools for a full build.

↑ The Sprinter van is beloved by home-converters the world over for its ubiquity, space and tough mechanicals.

For an in-depth discussion on building a motorhome yourself, including very detailed information on the legalities and regulations governing conversions for insurance and registration purposes, the *Build Your Own Motorcaravan* manual from Haynes is a great place to start, if we do say so ourselves.

The big downside to this approach is that even the best DIY home-build van will struggle to be worth as much as the van it is based on. So, while building your own vehicle or buying someone else's project is a great way to get a foot on the ladder, it is a riskier prospect if you need to get your money back later on.

The easiest way to sidestep that of course is to hang on to the van and keep using it. If you have no plans to sell, then the lower resale price isn't an issue.

DIY for van lifers

Even if you don't consider yourself a very 'DIY' person, having a basic awareness of your van and how it is hanging together is a great idea. Carrying out a basic survey of the van every six months or so will help to ensure that you are aware of what is deteriorating, what is urgent and what can be left for another year. Plainly, this is less of an issue with newer vans, but vigilance when it comes to spotting hanging cables, pipes or unforeseen damage will all save grief later on, no matter how much you spent on the van itself.

A survey of your motorhome when you first get it will allow you to build a picture of tasks that require attention. Spend a morning going around the van, making notes, taking photos and looking for evidence of future failure. You don't need to be a mechanic to do this. If there is oil on the floor under the engine, a rusty brake disc or

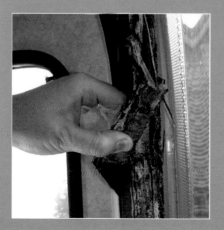

↓ Pretty much anything can be fixed, even damp frames which crumble away when you look at them...

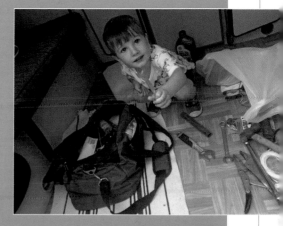

↑ Get the family involved in the DIY projects. It could be handy to have more than one person who knows their way around the spanners.

the horn only works every third push, take note. Also pay attention to rust, however minor it appears. You don't have to be able to fix it, but noticing it and getting it looked at by someone who can could prevent problems in the future.

It's likely that you'll notice all manner of minor issues, such as a cloudy window, cosmetic rust or a sticky door latch. None will stop you from using the van and none represents a safety issue, and fixing them all at the same time would be expensive or lay the van up. Instead, grade the problems in terms of severity. The most urgent can be attended to first, others can be left until the winter, next year or even indefinitely if they don't worry you.

Knowing your van well will ensure regular maintenance and repairs can be planned and budgeted for. This minimises the chances of a breakdown and ensures that, through a process of gradual improvement, your van gets better with age.

Case study

Humans **David Howells**
Vehicle **2009 Mercedes Sprinter**

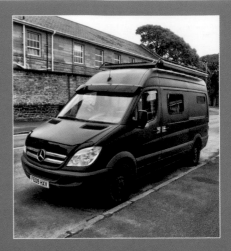

David Howells wanted a specific vehicle for a specific task but a look around what was on the market showed that there was nothing which quite fitted the brief.

David had a plan to climb the highest peaks in every country in Europe, and a van is the ideal way to travel between the peaks and a great place to recover after a day or two ascended a mountain. David wanted a van which could enable some wild,'off-grid' camping, big enough to be comfortable and with a proper bed, but small enough to slip along mountain passes and park up discreetly.

While no off-the-peg vans fitted the bill, David did find a self-build that looked promising. It was a Mercedes Sprinter in good mechanical shape which had a basic conversion completed by the vendor.

'I bought it from a guy called Adam Cooper who is a surfer and a carpenter. He built a good quality interior but it was basic. He had a two-burner hob, a bed and some lights which is all you need a for a night or two by the beach. I didn't want to start pulling apart what he'd done, so when I go the van, I started

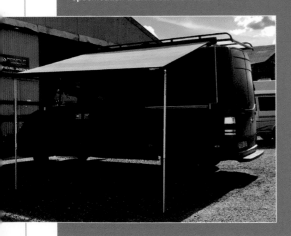

⬇ David's van was someone else's self-build, which he has steadily improved to the specification that meets his needs.

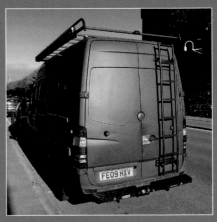

⬇ External upgrades include solar panels, roofracks and ladders to ensure David can carry everything he needs when exploring.

planning a few upgrades which would allow me to do what I need'.

To support David's mountain mission, he added a pair of 200w solar panels to charge his twin leisure batteries and an inverter. This allows him to keep laptops, phones and all other gadgets charged as he goes.

For comfort, he added a gas heater and a pair of fridges. While doing this, he opted for new oak worktops, ladders, steps and a roof rack to help with storage issues and had the engine remapped to give a little more power for climbing those European hills.

David says the van cost around £17,000 and a further £10,000 has been spent to convert it into the vehicle that he now owns - a bespoke light expedition vehicle which ticks all the boxes for him.

David is very honest about the van and says that he still has some concerns.

'It's great for what I am going to use it for, but it's not perfect. There is no air-con, and no fans or ventilation as such. In extreme heat it will get very hot. This wasn't a conscious decision, the solar array and roof box, and interior work by a previous owner, mean there is no roof space for a vent. Being painted black won't help either. I'll see how I get on.'

It's not just the heat that might cause problems. 'If it gets extremely cold, I could have an issue too. The inside is insulated, but with no front partition between the cab and the living area, I need to keep an eye on the temperature inside. I'm aware of it all and it's my choice so I don't mind a bit. For 90% of the time it will do me perfectly, exactly as it is.'

→ The interior is plush and cosy, but the vast, practical storage area under the bed is what will make the van liveable in.

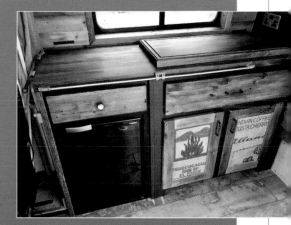

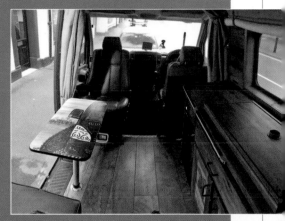

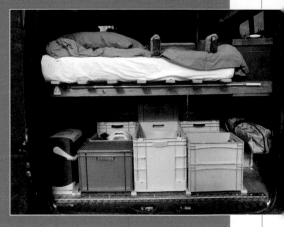

Detailed buyers' guides

There are a lot of commercial vehicles on the market, and we can't cover them all, so we've concentrated on the ones that you'll find the most motorcaravans based on, or the ones that are finding favour with the self-building scene.

We've also omitted the most modern stuff. The current crop of Fiat/Peugeot, Vauxhall/Renault, Volkswagen and Mercedes are modern enough that they should be in excellent health. If they aren't, go and find another one. We've concentrated on models that are getting on a bit as they are the easiest ones to unwittingly get wrong.

We've covered many of the most popular vans you'll find on the market here, but eBay, Gumtree and Preloved are full of other types of van, too. Some are ripe for conversion while others are ready for adventure. Availability on its own is not a good enough reason to buy, though.

Regardless of the vehicle you choose, it goes without saying that a good example is better than a bad one. This is obvious enough, but in most cases, good examples of less desirable vehicles are a better bet than a soggy example of something more fashionable.

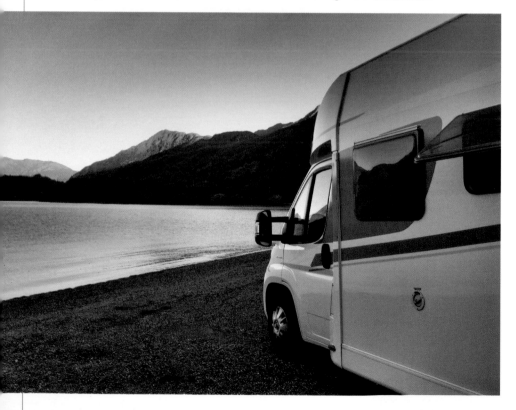

Running costs

Working out how much to set aside for running an older van can be a bit of a struggle, but in general these ongoing costs will be high compared with those of a new van. That said, the total amount will still be considerably less than the sum you'll lose thanks to depreciation if you buy a new one.

When running an older vehicle, set money aside to cover the cost of unexpected repairs. As a general rule, £500 will keep a van serviced and £1,000 will fix pretty much anything mechanical on an older vehicle. It won't buy a new engine or gearbox, but it should be enough to buy a good second-hand unit or to have yours rebuilt if it starts to suffer.

Such big repairs are rare, however, unless you are very unlucky. The main expense is the ongoing maintenance. Again, this fits the housing analogy well.

You would call in a techncian if your washing machine became a bit noisy or didn't do a very good job of cleaning – you wouldn't wait for it to catch fire before calling in help. Treat a van the same way. If it is becoming harder to stop or start or there is a new noise, get it looked at before it leaves you stranded or empties your bank account, or possibly both.

Most older commercial vehicles are fairly straightforward to work on, so a good general mechanic will be able to handle most servicing tasks, and motorhome workshops will tackle any other repairs. Avoid the huge aircraft hangar dealer sites if you have an older truck, though. Instead, find a good independent or mobile service agent to ensure that your van is kept in good shape, for which you'll pay an amount more commensurate with the value of the vehicle.

⬇ Modern vans are only more reliable than their older counterparts if they are kept serviced, even if the mileage covered is small.

⬇ Expect older vans to need the occasional big repair, alongside the basic maintenance. It's a good idea to budget for this.

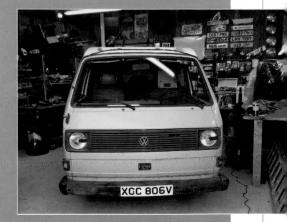

Detailed buyers' guide
Fiat Ducato Mk1

Spotter's guide

Later models have an upgraded cab and a few improvements to details. The easiest way to spot them is to look at the cab doors. Early-model cab windows are horizontal, while facelift ones slope downwards. Fiat, Peugeot and Talbot models can be told apart by the front grilles, but mechanically they are identical.

Brief history

A collaboration between Peugeot, Citroën and Fiat, the Fiat Ducato Mk1 was the predecessor to the current Fiat/Peugeot X250 model that underpins the majority of the European motorhome market. At launch, it immediately found favour with converters due to it being front-wheel drive, affordable and flexible. Most right-hand drive models were badged as Talbot Express.

Instant expert

If you are shopping with a relatively modest budget, you will inevitably end up looking

Spec Box

YEARS IN PRODUCTION 1981–1993
ALSO KNOWN AS Talbot Express (UK only); Peugeot J5; Citroën C25 and Alfa Romeo AR6 (sold in France and Italy respectively)
ENGINE TYPES 2.0-litre petrol; 1.9-litre diesel; 2.5-litre diesel; 2.5-litre turbo-diesel

at a selection of rolling homes based on the variously named versions of the Mk1 Fiat Ducato. It dominated the market for coachbuilt motorhome chassis during its life, but with even the newest now being at least 25 years old, they are firmly in budget territory.

Given their age, corrosion is the major consideration. Windscreen surrounds are very prone to rot, as are the door steps, wheel arches and wings. A good bodyshop can repair pretty much anything you'll find, but this isn't cheap.

None could be described as fast, but the best performer is the turbo-diesel model. The other diesels all work hard, but it is imperative that they are serviced regularly. On a test drive, be very wary of starting difficulties and low coolant levels. The former can be a simple glow plug issue but then again it could be more serious. Low coolant can point to cylinder issues, which are expensive to resolve. Don't worry about the diesels looking a bit oily – they all do. In fact, be suspicious if they don't.

The single petrol engine is a bit weedy, but it is reassuringly simple and has few vices. Rough running is likely to be due to a failing fuel pump or because the vehicle is in need of a good service. Throaty noises are caused by damaged exhaust manifolds and this is usually the result of failing engine mounts. These are fiddly fixes, but not particularly expensive if you can get hold of the parts.

The gear change deserves special mention. Left-hand-drive models have a

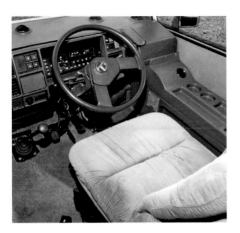

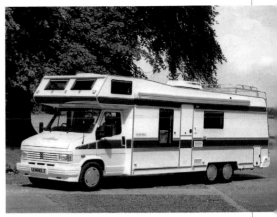

↑ The cab is basic by modern standards. Take a test drive to ensure you are comfortable driving it.

↑ Mk1 Ducato and Talbot coachbuilts come in all shapes and sizes. Look out for damp or rust.

snicky column-shift gear change, whether an automatic or manual gearbox is fitted. Automatic gearboxes were never offered in the UK, so right-hand-drive ones have a ponderous floor-mounted manual change to contend with, which takes some getting used to.

If gear selection is really difficult, new engine mounts may help. The rear-most one in particular supports the whole back of the engine when it wears, making gears hard to find. If you find the gears but the gear lever feels like you are stirring porridge and you keep punching the dashboard, this may be something that can be adjusted. The gear linkage is complex, but a patient garage or owner will be able to improve things. Don't expect sports car gear changes, though, however much you adjust.

Other than that, the only things left to worry about are the brakes and suspension, but those are pretty basic and service items such as rubber bushes, brake discs and pads are available from your local parts counter.

Verdict

There is great value to be had if you are looking at vehicles based on the various versions of the original Fiat Ducato. A lot depends on the conversion, but if you can find one that has had any rust issues sorted and that's in good mechanical health, you'll have a great motorhome.

Expert tips

- If the clutch is heavy or the speedo is very wobbly, check the cables aren't snagged or cable tied together under the bonnet.
- Headlights are a common MOT failure point. Budget a couple of hundred pounds for replacements if the silvering has disappeared.
- Saggy rear suspension is common, even in vehicles in good condition. Aftermarket spring assisters can straighten things up for sensible money.

Detailed buyers' guide
Fiat Ducato X230/X240

Spotter's guide

X230 models have smaller headlights and there is no front grille and 'concertina-style' bellows on the wing mirror arms. X244 models from around 2003 onwards have larger headlamps, separated by a radiator grille, solid plastic mirror arms and a host of detail upgrades.

Brief history

The X230 Ducato, Boxer and Relay models replaced the Mk1 Ducato and J5 in 1993 and were a substantial improvement. Many of the things that had made the earlier model popular with converters remained in place, such as the low floors, flexible platform and competitive pricing, but now with stronger mechanicals and more contemporary styling.

Instant expert

You are very unlikely to find anything other than a diesel engine in one of these vans. Earlier models had a choice of a 1.9-litre

Spec Box

YEARS IN PRODUCTION 1993–2006
ALSO KNOWN AS Peugeot Boxer; Citroën Relay
ENGINE TYPES 1.9-litre diesel; 1.9-litre turbo-diesel; 2.5-litre diesel; 2.5-litre turbo-diesel

diesel in turbo and non-turbo form, with bigger 2.5- and 2.8-litre diesels reserved for larger vehicles.

It's likely that you'll observe some oil around the engine bay, but be wary of obviously 'wet' engines. Starting issues and smoke are the big warning signs of impending sickness. Broadly though, these are pretty tough units.

With the facelift in 2003/04, more powerful common-rail units came along in 2.0-litre non-intercooled turbo-diesel, and 2.3- or 2.8-litre intercooled turbo-diesels.

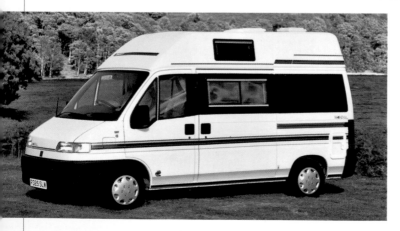

← When looking at high-top models, inspect the sills and wheelarches for rust.

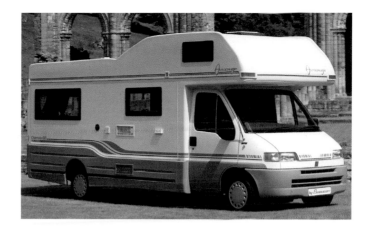

→ All versions are pretty tough mechanically, but big coachbuilts ask a lot of the engines. A test drive is a must to verify the van's health.

These were a considerable upgrade on the earlier models, offering smoother power delivery without any reliability penalty. As with most modern diesels, excessive smoke when accelerating indicates turbo issues, while poor performance and starting maladies speak of diesel pump and injector issues, which are expensive to solve.

All right-hand-drive models had five-speed manual gearboxes and these can give issues, particularly with regard to fifth gear. Walk away if you can't get fifth gear, or budget for a swap.

Aside from weird electrical issues, these are good vans. The main enemy is likely to be lack of use. Brakes in particular do not like inactivity, so ensure the handbrake works, and look for evidence of rusty brake discs after a run around the block. Drum brakes, where fitted, can seize, too. Noisy wheel bearings are common in vans that have been laid up, so listen for the telltale rumble on your test drive.

These vans are fairly rust-resistant, certainly compared to the earlier models, but age is against them now so pay careful attention to the front crossmember and the right-hand chassis leg, which can both collect water. The crossmember can be replaced fairly easily but changing the chassis leg is very involved work.

Verdict

These are absolutely excellent vans as a motorhome base vehicle. Ensure they get used regularly, don't be too rough with the interior trim and keep on top of the maintenance and you will have a great vehicle. Later ones drive better but the earlier ones have simpler technology. Get the best you can find.

Expert tips

- A drainpipe from the base of the windscreen should run down inside the engine bay and exit near the gear linkage. If it runs incorrectly, water can contaminate the gearbox oil and cost you a lot of cash.
- Low coolant can often be traced to a weeping radiator. This is cheap and simple to fix. A wrecked engine due to overheating is not. Don't top up without investigating.

Detailed buyers' guide
Mazda Bongo Friendee

Spotter's guide

The engine position means that cab seats cannot swivel. Adverts stating 'AFT' mean the van has the Mazda factory roof. Facelift models have deeper headlamps, a larger front grill, and different rear lights.

Brief history

The Bongo Friendee launched in 1995 as an eight-seater MPV and for the Japanese market. It was also sold as the Ford Freda but broadly the two were identical. It wasn't until the early 2000s that they started arriving in the UK as imported second-hand vehicles and they quickly found a niche as affordable alternatives to elderly Volkswagens and expensive new campers.

Instant expert

In the early 2000s, finding an affordable used campervan was very difficult. The options were to buy new or get an ageing Volkswagen and put up with ongoing maintenance, and this was why imports from Japan became popular. Enterprising UK dealers realised that a good source of well-equipped right-hand-drive vehicles

existed in Japan, so they started importing them in the form of the Bongo Friendee.

As standard, they were eight-seater MPVs with seating that folded to make a double bed. Some had simple kitchens installed from the factory and many had the electrically powered 'Auto Free Top' elevating roof. As well as giving these little vans good headroom, this feature made them into a simple four-berth camper. Their standard air-conditioning, automatic gearboxes and electronic window blinds were all very rare options in UK campers, so they were an immediate hit.

Mechanically, it is a fairly simple line-up. There are three engines: two petrol and one diesel. Most had automatic gearboxes and models were labelled as SGL3 for two-wheel drive, or SGL5 for all-wheel-drive.

Buyers are mainly looking for mechanical issues to be wary of. Head gasket failure is the most serious of these. Check the coolant reservoir under the bonnet for evidence of oil contamination. Further evidence is uncovered by checking under the engine oil filler caps. They are accessed by looking under the driver's seat (diesel) or passenger seat (petrol). If the contents appear more like pancake mix than engine oil, expensive investigations await.

If that is all looking good, listen for odd clonks and bangs on your test drive, which are likely to be down to worn suspension. This is not expensive to fix, but certainly something to use to negotiate down the price. Noisy or ineffective brakes are

---

Spec Box

YEARS IN PRODUCTION 1995–2005
ALSO KNOWN AS Ford Freda
ENGINE TYPES 2.0-litre four-cylinder petrol; 2.5-litre V6 petrol; 2.5-litre turbo-diesel

common in vans that don't move very often, so try the handbrake on your test drive. Again, it's not an expensive fix, but it will cost you at MOT time. The final test is to wind the steering from side to side. Inconsistent weighting and noise suggest a new steering rack is on the cards – another common Bongo black mark.

Despite their relative youth, Bongos do suffer from rust issues, mostly because Mazda was not expecting them to contend with UK winters. The rear wheel arches are usually the first place where you'll find telltale bubbles under the paint and that is a sure sign that all is not well. The sills – the metalwork running between the wheels at ground level – can also get messy, so look for evidence of holes, scabs or hasty patch-ups.

Sliding door difficulties are often due to little more than lack of lubrication, but do pay attention to the electric elevating roof. It should raise and lower smoothly and quickly.

Living in the Mazda Bongo

Comfort depends on the sort of conversion your Bongo has. For weekends, one of the many conversions utilising the standard MPV seating as the bed will probably be fine. If you are planning longer excursions, however, you might want to hunt for a more traditional conversion with a VW-style rock and roll bed, as they give you a flatter bed and better storage. In all cases, the Bongo is a small vehicle, so check you can get comfy both behind the wheel and in the cabin.

Verdict

A Bongo Friendee answers a lot of campervan questions for a lot of people. It has enough cab comforts to be

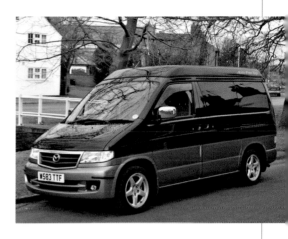

⬆ Very practical and useful as a camper you can live with every day, most Bongos are well-kitted out too.

considered a usable everyday vehicle, but is a capable enough camping vehicle to take away for an extended break. A diesel four-wheel-drive model with an automatic gearbox and a good-quality camper conversion makes a great first introduction to van life.

Expert tips

- If the handbrake isn't working well, look for evidence of oil around the back wheels. A failed seal can coat the rear brakes in oil and that is a tricky fix.
- Head gasket problems are often caused by low coolant levels. When checking the coolant reservoir, if the level looks low, suspect a leak. The chief suspect is the top engine coolant house, which often shows signs of cracking or expansion when it is on its last legs. If it springs a leak, it can cause a head gasket failure.

Detailed buyers' guide
Volkswagen Transporter T3

Spotter's guide

Very early models have metal air intakes at the back, rather than the later plastic ones.

All diesels and water-cooled petrols have a second grille under the main one. Four-wheel-drive 'Syncro' models are highly-prized as off-road campers, and command a hefty price premium.

Brief history

The Transporter T3 was an all-new vehicle that replaced the much-loved but ancient T2 in 1980. Although the rear-engined configuration was carried over from the T2, very little else was. Early models were fairly crudely equipped, but later models were available with power steering, plusher interiors, electric windows and mirrors, and many other little treats.

Instant expert

While the T3 has little in common mechanically with the T2 that it replaced, a lot of the buying advice is transferable. Unless you like to spend your weekends

welding, or paying someone else to, rust is the big enemy.

The sides of these vans are criss-crossed with seams, which are where the panels were welded together and the gaps were filled with flexible sealant at the factory. Some 30 years later, the sealant has often dried out, which allows rust to start to take hold. It is fairly easy to spot, unless an unscrupulous seller has covered it up to inflate the price.

In terms of severity, you want to check the sills for obvious rust or evidence of patch-up repairs. The area in front of the back wheels is prone to corrosion and is where the rear suspension mounts to the body, so any tin worm here is serious. Check immediately behind the front wheels, at the bottom of the B-pillar and in areas where years of road muck can accumulate and start to eat away at the steel.

Parts are available to fix all of this, but it is expensive, time-consuming work. Rust around the windscreen is common and will cause water leaks into the cab area and encourage rust in the cab floor. Also check around the roof gutters on high-roof and elevating-roof vans. Gutter repairs are tricky. Tailgates and doors do rust but these are less serious issues as these aren't structurally significant areas. That said, it doesn't make repairs any cheaper.

When making mechanical checks, it makes sense to have someone with you who knows something about the oily bits. Brakes and suspension usually cause few problems, aside from the hefty trailing

Spec Box

YEARS IN PRODUCTION 1980–1991
ALSO KNOWN AS T25; Wedge; Brick; Vanagon; Caravelle; Microbus
ENGINE TYPES 1.6-litre, 2.0-litre air-cooled petrol; 1.9-litre, 2.1-litre water-cooled petrol; 1.6-litre, 1.7-litre diesel; 1.6-litre turbo-diesel

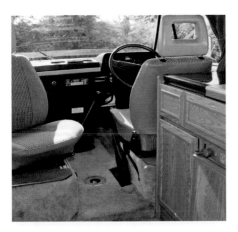

↑ Professional interior conversions such as this Auto Sleeper remain very desirable, if a little dated.

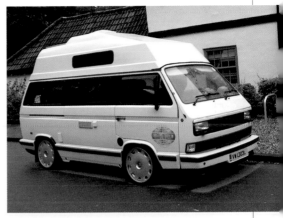

↑ VW fans are very keen on modifications, and there are loads of off-the-shelf upgrades available.

arms at the back of the van, which can rust and eventually collapse.

Engine-wise, though, you need to have your wits about you. The air-cooled engines are the simplest to use and maintain. Water-cooled petrols are more powerful and more refined but coolant leaks, overheating and exhaust issues all indicate expensive headaches. Look for evidence of servicing or proper repairs to ease your angst. The non-turbo-diesels are tough but fairly terrible, while the little 1.6-litre turbo-diesel offers a fraction more oomph. In the case of all engines, however, if they are smothered in oil, smoky or difficult to start, then budget for bills.

To get over the many engine issues, modern engine swaps are fairly common. Installation of a more modern 1.9TDi or 1.8-litre petrol engine boosts reliability if done well. And adding a Subaru flat-four engine can give a hot hatch a scare. In the case of these conversions, though, ask to see receipts for the work as unpicking someone's home-made project can cause real heartache.

Verdict

If you want a practical camper and don't mind the reliability foibles of a classic car, the T3 makes a good choice. It isn't a cheap option, but great spares support, a huge community and a modern retro look make them a desirable base vehicle. An early Westfalia Joker with the 2.0-litre air-cooled petrol engine and no serious rust is a hugely desirable vehicle.

Expert tips

- On water-cooled models, check the heater works. Replacing the blower switch isn't too hard, but changing the heater motor requires the dashboard to be removed and is a horrid job. If the heater doesn't get hot, it could indicate cooling issues that are tricky to fix. Beware.
- A modern electric power-steering conversion makes a huge difference to the way they drive.

Is a T2 Transporter the perfect camper?

There is no vehicle more closely associated with the idea of living in a van than the Volkswagen Transporter, particularly the T2 or Bay Window model that was made between 1967 and 1979.

The T2 Transporter replaced the narrower T1 but, crucially, improved on it in almost every way. It was an immediate hit and that early popularity has never really waned. The German-built models ceased production in 1979, but the modified T2C versions remained in production until 2016 in Brazil, where they are a common sight. A reasonable number were brought to the UK by Danbury and were sold new until 2017.

↓ The T2 cabin is pretty basic, whether you are looking at an original, or a continuation model such as this one.

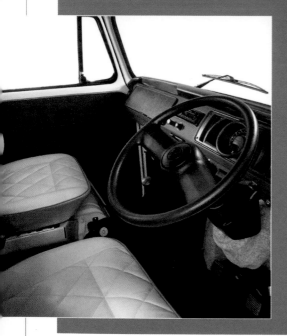

There is little question that the T2 is a great-looking vehicle, and with a good conversion, they are a lovely camper, for shorter sojourns at least. Before setting your heart on one, however, you must know what you are getting into. They are old vehicles, so you cannot expect modern road manners, reliability or comfort, despite paying a price that feels like these should be on offer.

Even rough ones cost a lot of money and they are likely to cost you a lot more than that to put straight. Rust breaks out everywhere and many owners have their hearts broken by the seemingly endless spending on repairs. Unless you have the skills to tackle the problems yourself, you really should beware of buying a project.

If you still want a T2, then buy one, but go into it with your eyes open and don't be blinded by shiny paint and bunting. Bargains always turn into money pits. Spend the money, buy a nice one and enjoy it.

Alternatively, get the looks with a bit more modernity by finding a modern Danbury T2C. You won't have the rust or unreliability to contend with, but you'll still have classic car brakes and heavy steering to temper your fun.

If travel is more of a priority than platform, there are shrewder ways to spend. An excellent VW T3 costs half of what an equivalent T2 would, still has plenty of VW scene credibility and is a far more usable vehicle. Put your head before your heart, though, and a T4 or T5 will give you reliability and access to the Vee-Dub show circuit with little of the heartache.

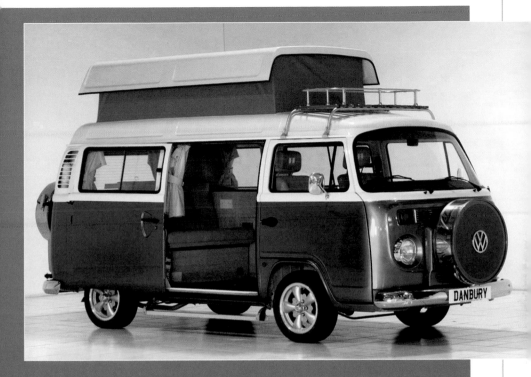

⬆ This is as modern a version of the T2 as you will find. Undoubtedly pretty, but make sure you can cope with the antiquated drive before buying one.

⬇ Bay window Type 2s come in two flavours. Early Bays (right) from 1967 on are felt to be prettiest, while Late Bays from 1973 on (left) have better engines, brakes and a host of other improvements.

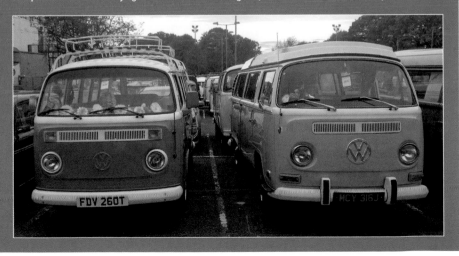

Detailed buyers' guide
Volkswagen Transporter T4

Spotter's guide

There are two versions of the T4 – referred to as the short-nose and the long-nose. The long-nose version was introduced in 1996 to provide room for the V6 petrol engine, but the very last TDi models in 2002/03 also got the restyled nose. It is much more common in left-hand drive models.

Brief history

The T4 is considered by many in the VW scene to be the last of the proper 'old school' Volkswagens. Given that they are more rust-resistant and less prone to problems than earlier ones, that seems a bit unfair. A T4 is a far more enticing prospect for those who want to hit the road without a toolkit in tow.

⬇ Longnose versions of the T4 are characterised by the slanted headlamps. They are rare as UK vehicles, but desirable.

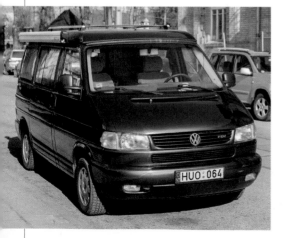

Instant expert

The T4 is new enough to avoid some issues but old enough to retain others, so you need to keep your wits about you when buying. On the bright side, compared to older VWs, it's far easier to find a good one. The T4 is far better at resisting corrosion than earlier campers, so while you should be vigilant in looking for tin worm, you don't need to fret to quite the same extent. Post-1996 facelift models are better than earlier ones.

When looking at a prospect, concentrate low down. The sills that run between the front and back wheels get the most thrown at them on the road, and on long-wheelbase models in particular are prone to receiving a clout on uneven ground. The ends are particularly keen to rust. Have a good look at the rear wheel arches while you're there, too, as well as the cab door steps. If you lift the bonnet you'll get to see the base of the windscreen surround panel and the inner wings, neither of which are immune to rust.

You should also check the major panels for rust – the cab doors are generally

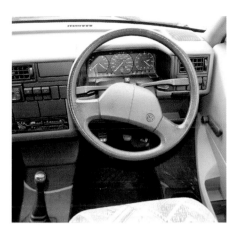

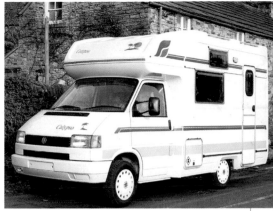

↑ The cabin is simple but everything will likely still work properly. Power steering is a huge plus.

↑ Coachbuilt T4s are rare, and tend to look a little ungainly, but they make a lovely van.

unscathed, but the side door can rust and the tailgate models can leak, letting rust take hold in the back of the van.

Given the age of the vans, you are much better off looking for models that are in good condition, rather than ones with specific engines. That said, be excited if you find either of the turbo-diesels. The smaller 1.9-litre is simple if slower, while the larger 2.5TDI is smoother but more complicated. The other diesels are sluggish and the 2.4-litre one has a reputation for head gasket problems too, so check the coolant level if you're looking at one. The VR6 petrol is very rare but highly prized. The other petrols are relatively trouble-free, provided that they are looked after.

On a test drive, listen for clunks from the front suspension, which could indicate either ball joints or suspension bushes need to be replaced. This is not serious, but it's worth asking for a few quid off the asking price to cover the replacements. If the van is difficult to get into gear or jumps out of gear, however, that is a red flag and

indicates that a replacement gearbox is needed. The other thing to look out for is electrical issues. Check that central locking, road lights and the ignition switch all work properly.

Verdict

In many ways, the T4 is the sweet spot of the VW line-up. You sidestep many of the rust and reliability concerns of the older vans, but you don't have the complexity and cost associated with the newest. Buy well and you'll have a van to take you anywhere.

Expert tips

- Early models didn't have power steering. Take a test drive to ensure you can manage driving them.
- Check for clutch fluid leaks above the pedals box, which are common. It is an early warning that you might end up without a clutch sometime soon.

Detailed buyers' guide
Volkswagen Transporter T5

Spotter's guide

There are two body lengths: short and long wheelbase. Semi- and high-roof models are rare. Facelift models have three-spoke steering wheels and the headlights touch the ends of the grille.

Brief history

The Transporter T5 was launched in 2004 to replace the T4, but was a big step forwards in every way from the earlier models. It retained a reputation as one of the more car-like commercials to drive but was bigger in every dimension and a step up in quality. It was replaced by the very similar-looking T6 in 2015.

Instant expert

Unlike most other manufacturers, Volkswagen offer a factory-sanctioned range of camper conversions under the name 'California'. These aren't especially plush conversions, but they are very nicely put together and guaranteed to hold their value. There are also hundreds of third-party conversions to choose from from dozens of manufacturers, and a

peerless marketplace of parts for those who want to convert their own. You won't struggle to find a T5 camper.

The hard bit is sifting the good from the indifferent conversions. The California is arguably the best of the three, followed by vans made by the top-tier converters such as Auto-Sleepers, Bilbo's and Reimo. Thereafter, there are a lot of excellent conversions from smaller manufacturers, but once they are a couple of years old, it can be hard to tell a good one from something overpriced and underwhelming. It's difficult to give general advice, but look inside the cabinets and underneath the drawers to see whether it looks like it has been thrown together, or whether it seems nicely made. Use your ears on a test drive, too. If you hear a lot of clatter and noise, this is an indicator of a lower-quality conversion.

Buying the actual van is considerably easier. There are two periods of build for the T5. The original T5 was offered from 2004 with a four-cylinder 1.9-litre turbo-diesel with a five-speed gearbox and a choice of two outputs – 84PS and 102PS. An Audi-sourced five-cylinder 2.5-litre diesel was also offered with 131PS or 174PS and a six-speed gearbox.

There was a substantial facelift in 2009 that redesigned the front and rear ends of the van and simplified the engine line-up. The so-called T5.1 range all had 2.0-litre turbo-diesels in four different outputs.

It is very commonplace for owners to uprate the lower-output engines. A simple

Spec Box

YEARS IN PRODUCTION 2004–2015
ALSO KNOWN AS T5.1; T26; T28; T30; T32
ENGINE TYPES 1.9-litre turbo-diesel; 2.5-litre turbo-diesel; 2.0-litre turbo-diesel

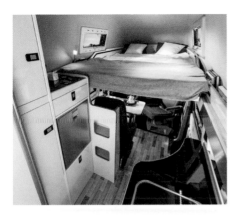

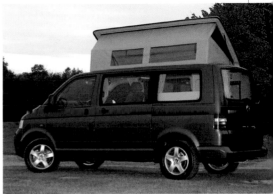

↑ High-top T5s like this Club Joker offer huge space and still drive very well, despite looking top-heavy.

↑ A T5 blends affordability with usability, but if you want a posh factory conversion, budget for £30k plus.

electronic update costing a few hundred pounds is all that is needed and it can transform a weedy engine into something more muscular. The only mechanical differences between the high- and low-output engines are the gearboxes, with the lower ones having only five gears.

When buying, there are relatively few mechanical issues to beware of and those that do exist centre around the clutches and gearboxes. An illuminated engine warning light indicates another common issue: a failed exhaust gas recirculation valve. Other than that, listening for suspension clanks and bangs on the test drive is the main caution to exercise, but repairs are not beyond a good home mechanic.

T5s have a reputation for hoovering up the miles, so provided that there is evidence of regular servicing, high mileages should not be a concern. One thing that you should not have to contend with is rust. The oldest T5s are now approaching their 15th birthday but they are very well protected against rust, unlike most of their forebears.

Verdict

For those looking for their first taste of van life, a T5 offers the easiest introduction. Short-wheelbase versions are not much longer than an estate car, or very different to drive, and the range of conversions available means that there genuinely is something for everyone. The biggest barrier is cost. All official conversions cling on to their value tenaciously.

Expert tips

- Owners love to personalise their Transporters. Avoid heavily modified ones unless that is what you are after. Crude suspension mods and huge wheels are very popular in the VW scene but they rarely improve the way they drive.
- Tailgate models are more popular for motorhome conversion than the rear twin-doors. You can convert to a tailgate if you can't find the van you want.

Detailed buyers' guide
Bedford CF/CF2

Bedford's venerable CF was a camper and coachbuilt base vehicle throughout its life. It was a very simple vehicle, built around a separate chassis and a basic drivetrain, but it isn't without its quirks. The engine sat between the driver and passenger, much like it does in a truck, making for a characteristic driving position.

Some parts are scarce, particularly body panels for early models, and the combined front wheel arch/A-post assembly will vex even the most competent panel beater. Many mechanical parts are only available second-hand, too.

On a more positive note, farmyard simplicity means that a CF remains a viable

↓ CFs may soldier on forever mechanically, but rust repairs can be surprisingly tricky.

motorhome more than 30 years since the last ones left the factory. Petrol versions are more civilised than diesels and 2.3-litre models in particular are fairly quick, by the standards of the day.

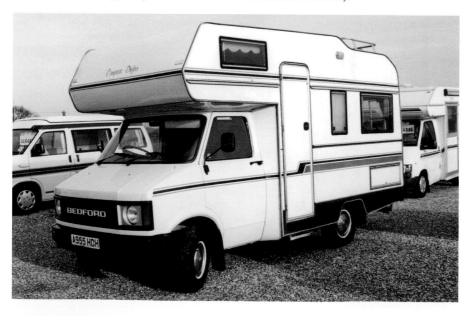

Classic campers

Some of the best-looking campers you'll find date from the 1960s and 70s. Cute styling, stripy roofs and handsome real-wood interiors make them tempting if you want to stand out.

If you're planning on staying fairly local, a classic offers good value compared to a modern motorhome. Vehicles based on the Commer or the Bedford CA look great, but they rely on very old technology and can give up at any moment. You could be waiting days for spare parts to arrive if you break down. On the plus side, simple technology means that you can often get things going again if you know where to look.

If this is a route you want to go down, you need to obtain some basic mechanical skills to prevent yourself from being on first-name terms with the AA patrolman.

Typical faults relate to fuel, cooling and engine electrical problems, so if you know how to fit a set of points or clean out a carburettor, you'll be fine. Being able to adjust a drum brake is also a useful skill to have. If you are planning on trekking to the Continent, you should also replace all the rubber items in the fuel system in case you have to use ethanol-rich E10 petrol, which rots old rubber components.

If all this doesn't put you off, then you're a suitably sympathetic companion for a classic camper. The only other concession you need to make is time. Old vans are slow and low-geared compared to modern vehicles, so getting anywhere takes longer. If bouncing along B-roads and having constant conversations with admiring observers suits you, a classic might be perfect.

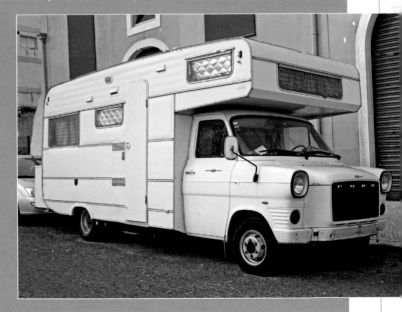

→ A well-sorted classic van will turn heads wherever you go but they simply cannot cover the ground like a modern truck.

Detailed buyers' guide
Ford Transit Mk1/2

The Ford Transit is tough, easy to fix and surprisingly civilised to drive, but they rot readily and rust is the main enemy. Owners have often swapped older coachbuilt bodies on to later chassis to overcome corrosion. Find a good one, though, and you might well have got a motorhome for life.

While Ford Transits don't attract the same manic pricing as older Volkswagens, Fords have fanatics of their own and prices tend towards the optimistic. However, this does mean that money spent on repairs is likely to reap rewards at resale time, compared with contemporary Bedfords or LDVs. Petrol models are more usable than the old York diesel-engined versions.

→ Pretty ancient now, but if the bodywork is good, consider taking one home.

⬇ As simple and as tough as teeth.

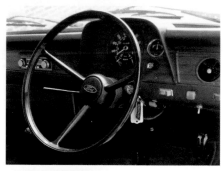

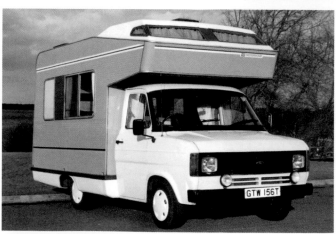

→ The Mk3 Transit is a cinch to work on and tough. They can rust everywhere though, so beware.

Detailed buyers' guide
Ford Transit Mk3

As with earlier incarnations of Ford's workhorse, the Mk3 was a class-leading drive but remained haunted by rust. Check everywhere for it if you are weighing up a purchase.

In common with older models, Mk3s were rear-wheel drive. That's good for traction, but makes the load area higher than those of rivals such as the Fiat Ducato and Volkswagen Transporter. This factor limited its appeal as a motorhome base during the 1990s, but there were some excellent conversions from the likes of Auto-Sleepers, among others, so it's worth a look if one comes up at the right price.

Facelift models from 1995–2000 have far nicer interior cabs and you may find the rare turbo-diesel model, which has a little extra oomph. The standard 2.5Di engines

are tough though and there is nothing wrong with them if oil changes and cambelt swaps are maintained. A non-rusty one is the aim. Everything else is fixable.

Top tips

- Best points: Tough mechanicals, good parts availability.
- Worst points: Rust.
- Try to find: Auto-Sleepers Frisky. The short-wheelbase Frisky is a flexible two-berth camper. The solid-sided elevating roof, heating and water systems mean it is well kitted out, but it's compact enough to be your daily driver. Highly desirable.

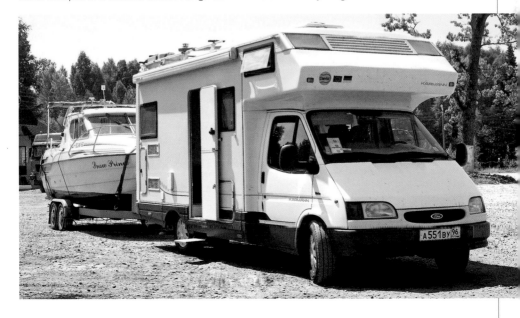

Walk-away faults for campervans and motorhomes

Terminal rust

Anything can be fixed, of course, but once a cheap camper or motorcaravan gets overtaken by rust, the route back to roadworthiness is long and littered with expense. Unless you are a competent welder, avoid vehicles with serious rust in structural areas.

Serious water ingress

Damp is a fact of life for older coachbuilts and you won't avoid it completely. In some, however, the damp may have spread too far, particularly if it results from porous body panels rather than localised damage.

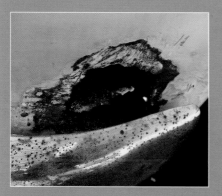

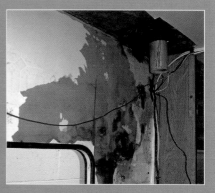

Crash damage

Getting body panels and mouldings for older coachbuilts is very tough. Unless you are happy to remodel and rebuild it yourself, accident-damaged coachbuilts are best left to the professionals.

Bodged VWs

Old Volkswagen buses rot and break down, but it doesn't stop people passing off complete rubbish as something worth buying. Don't pay over the odds for a project van just because of its badge.

Terrible self-builds

The definition of a self-build motorcaravan is pretty sketchy. Watch out for people chucking a mattress and a camping stove in a panel van, calling it a motorhome and adding 50 per cent to the asking price – eBay is full of them.

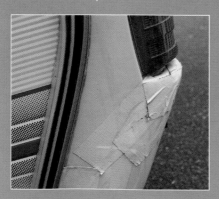

Detailed buyers' guide
Mercedes-Benz TN 'Bremen'

These old Mercedes vans are as tough as teeth and owners will regale you with stories of legendary reliability. Keep them talking, however, and they will also warn you that they are slow and prone to rust. If you happen upon a healthy one, though, it's worth stretching your budget to snap it up if possible.

The main thing that the TN had going for it was the size. The biggest versions were huge, with gross masses up to 4.6 tons, and caught the eye of some converters. The most common converter in the UK was Auto-Trail, who built a range of large, handsome coachbuilts on the TN platform. It was a popular base for European A-class coachbuilts too, with Hymer liking petrol-powered TNs as the basis of its flagship models.

In the UK, the only engines available were diesels. All were tough, but the later 2.4-litre diesels give you the best chance of keeping up with the traffic. By the time the TN went out of production, it was well off the pace of the similarly-sized Transit, but a

good one will be a more dependable truck.

If buying, look for evidence of balljoint replacement, kingpins being greased and regular services for the engine. All need doing frequently. If something does go wrong, parts availability from Mercedes is conspicuously good, pretty much anywhere in the world. Rust issues affecting the wings, doors and bonnet aren't a big worry but beware chassis or cab rust issues as they are tricky to treat.

➜ A legendarily tough platform for a motorhome. A good one is a fantastic, if slow, vehicle.

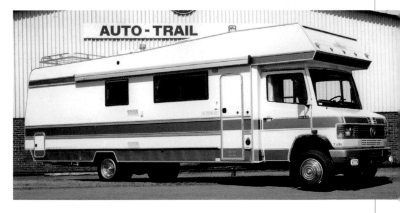

Detailed buyers' guide
Renault Trafic

The first-generation Renault Trafic was a lightweight, front-wheel drive commercial vehicle that proved popular with motorhome makers for a time. As with other front-wheel drive vans, the internal space is generous for the van's modest dimensions and that is one of the reasons why Auto-Sleepers, Elddis, Eriba and even Winnebago built on the platform.

As with a lot of older diesels, they are loud and not very powerful but they are not scared of work. Among the petrol models, aside from the weedy 1.4-litre lump, the others are smooth enough, quiet and capable, but fuel economy is fairly weak as all of them have to work hard to motivate a motorhome. Rust repairs are tricky due to the lightweight construction. The price on a fit one may be tempting. Invest in rust prevention.

Top tips

- Best points: Good to drive, mechanically simple.
- Worst points: Rust, some structural repairs are difficult.
- Try to find: Eriba Car. Pop-top coachbuilt motorhomes are a niche product but they have aged well. Like Eriba caravans, they were well made and beautifully packaged, but taller buyers should beware – headroom is limited.

⬇ The Renault Trafic is never going to be quick, but ones with stylish, high-quality coachbuilt conversions by the likes of Eriba remain desirable today as they age very well. Well worth seeking out.

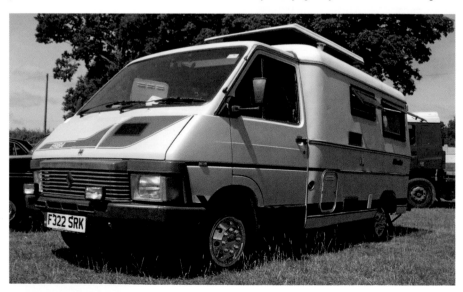

Case study

Human	**Jenny Owen**
Vehicle	**'Wilma' a 1980 VW T25 Transporter**

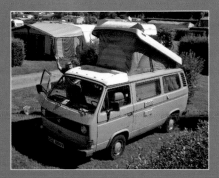

Jenny Owen had long wanted to own a camper, but says that her relationship with 'Wilma', her Volkswagen Transporter, has not always been an easy one.

'I've worked abroad for long periods in my role as a graphic designer but on my return to the UK from spells in the Far East, I was keen to see a bit more of the UK and Europe'.

'That was how I hit on the idea of a camper. Everyone was keen to tell me that Volkswagens cost a fortune, but with my boyfriend's help, we did a bit of research and decided that a "Type 25" offered an affordable route into getting a camper, but without the fragility of running a classic car. In truth, we weren't as clever as we thought!'

'We've travelled all over the UK and had a few forays across the Channel, but despite a promising papertrail of invoices and receipts, our van was pretty poorly when we acquired her. We've poured a fair few pounds and hundreds of hours into getting her more reliable and that is paying off now.'

'The VW scene is a mixture of styles and outlooks and some people love meeting up and chatting about the vans. We've done a few of those events and they are fun, but we mix it up a bit.'

'We are a bit more about the travel. We love heading off for a quiet break at an independent campsite or to a music festival. Even then, we prefer the more relaxed ones. Glastonbury is great, but for better value and ease of getting in and out, we've started going to some of the weirder ones. Cropredy Folk Festival and the Upton Blues Festival are so laid back and the van is the perfect base. I can't imagine going back to a tent now!'

'Ultimately, the places we go to are limited by the van as we have the smallest engine and we can't cover vast distances without weeks off work. That's fine at the moment. Getting behind the wheel and heading off for a few days is the best feeling though.'

'If my boyfriend is working, my sister will often come along. You can have a weekend away with a wander around a little town, a few glasses of wine and a barbecue for pennies if you have the van outside. I've certainly seen a lot more of the UK since getting Wilma!'

⬇ Jenny's VW is proving reliable at last, but unpicking years of neglect has been expensive.

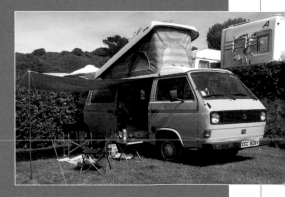

Should you go American?

Ask motorhome owners whether or not you should consider investing in an RV and you will likely hear sucking through teeth and lots of talk about terrible fuel economy and how they know someone who got one wedged between two villas in Spain and are still there now.

Scare stories are common, but common sense is often in shorter supply.

While it is fair to say they aren't for everyone, they can make a very sensible choice for certain buyers.

For people who wish to spend long periods in one or two sites over the winter, for instance, an RV is an excellent choice. Anything modern-ish will come with a television, air-conditioning, a generator, large waste and water tanks, and comfort as standard. They really are a different prospect from a European vehicle, with the emphasis on space, comfort and convenience, rather than lightweight camping simplicity. If you go for something that measures 25ft (7.6m)

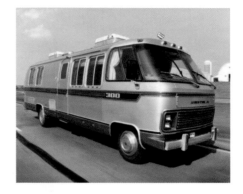

⬆ Airstream made a range of motorhomes, which look sensational but are rare in Europe.

⬇ The Winnebago Brave is what people typically picture when they think of an American RV.

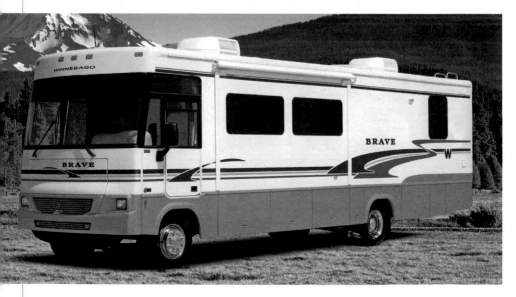

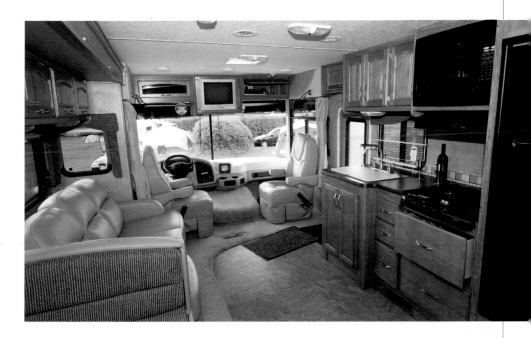

or less, you will be able to travel to most of the places that a Euro-coachbuilt will go, but you'll be more comfy.

There are obvious downsides. American RVs are left-hand drive, even the diesels like a drink, the largest ones are unusably huge, and all but the smallest require you to have either a pre-1997 driving licence or a C1 driving licence. Working out prices for older models is something of a lottery and spare parts supply can be patchy, too. At the very least, shipping parts from the USA can leave you off the road for longer than a Euro van would.

If you fancy an RV, start off by paying a visit to one of the specialist dealers dotted around the UK. Many operate hire services, so you can get behind the whool before committing, and they'll be able to advise on getting insurance, breakdown cover and other aspects of living your own American dream.

⬆ Any hassle on-road is compensated for by the vast interior on offer if you have a slide-out model.

⬇ Decorative finishes are typically a little dated for European tastes but kit-levels shame most houses.

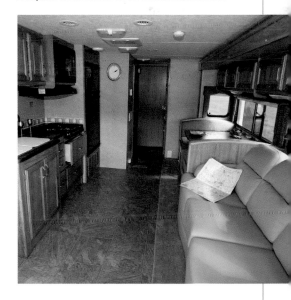

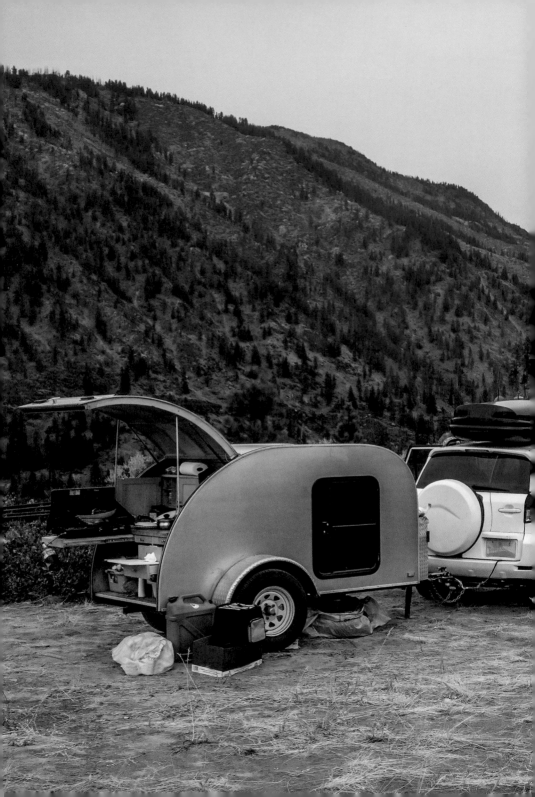

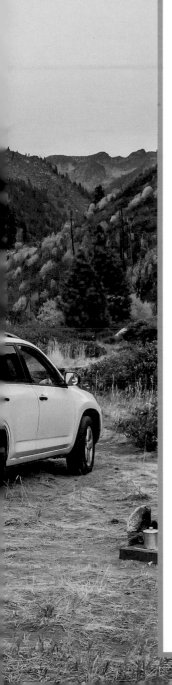

Chapter 4

Caravans and travel trailers

Compared to the world of campervans and motorhomes, caravans could not be easier to get your head around. They are simpler products and a great way to get your first taste of van life. Caravans do not conjure quite the same sun-blushed mental images of freedom and life on the open road, but if the aim is to sample lots of new places, cultures and histories, the means of getting there doesn't really make any difference. That the travel experience is different does not confer quality or value. Just preference.

What *is* a caravan?

We've established that caravans need towing to get anywhere, but that is only a good enough description to discern between a caravan and a motorhome. There is more to it.

Caravans don't have that many 'types' per se, but in the interests of making sure you know what you are looking at when you start hunting for one, we'll cover all towed leisure vehicles for the sake of completeness. Some caravans span more than one of the categories, but this is a useful guide.

Camping trailer

A camping trailer is a small trailer towed on wheels that you put your tent and other camping equipment in before heading off to a campsite. It forms no part of the accommodation.

Trailer tents

This is a very descriptive title. A trailer tent is typically a small trailer that forms part of the assembled structure of the tent on

Caravan blindness

This is a very real phenomenon afflicting visitors to caravan shows or large dealership forecourts: if you go in too many caravans, one after the other, you'll forget which ones you liked and which ones you didn't.

Try to form an idea about the key features (such as fixed bed, or maximum mass) you are looking for, and only go in the ones that fit your criteria. If you find things you like, use your camera phone to record details, taking pictures of the make and model. Avoid going in posh ones 'just to have a look' or ones that plainly aren't suitable or you'll go mad. Or, worse, buy the wrong one.

⬇ Folding campers are a great compromise between caravan comfort and the ease of towing a small trailer.

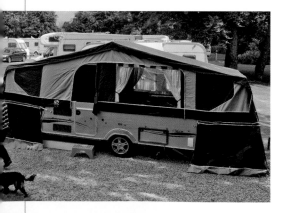

site. On arrival, you position the trailer on your pitch, unfold the structure and tension the canvas by pegging it to the ground. These structures are light, good value and an upgrade on a tent because, typically, you do not sleep on the floor – the beds are in the trailer. The trailers themselves are lightweight and many can be comfortably towed by any size of car, even the smallest.

Folding campers

This is quite nuanced, but the difference between a trailer tent and a folding camper is that you don't need to hammer anything into the ground before you use

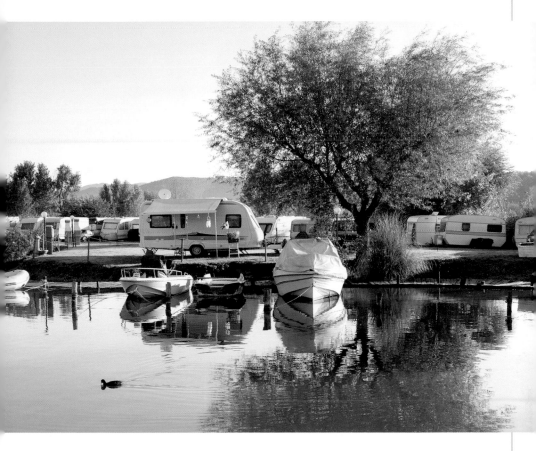

the latter. Some have solid sides, some have fabric sides, but both the beds and some form of living area are off the ground. The most common makes you'll find are Conway and Pennine.

⬆ Caravans need to be on a site. Wild camping is not really an option in most countries across Europe.

⬇ Trailer tents are an upgrade on a standard tent, but all that fabric needs looking after.

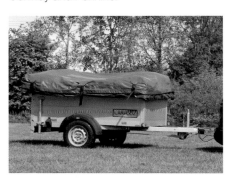

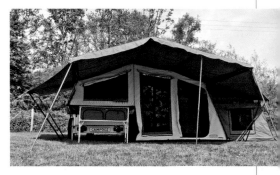

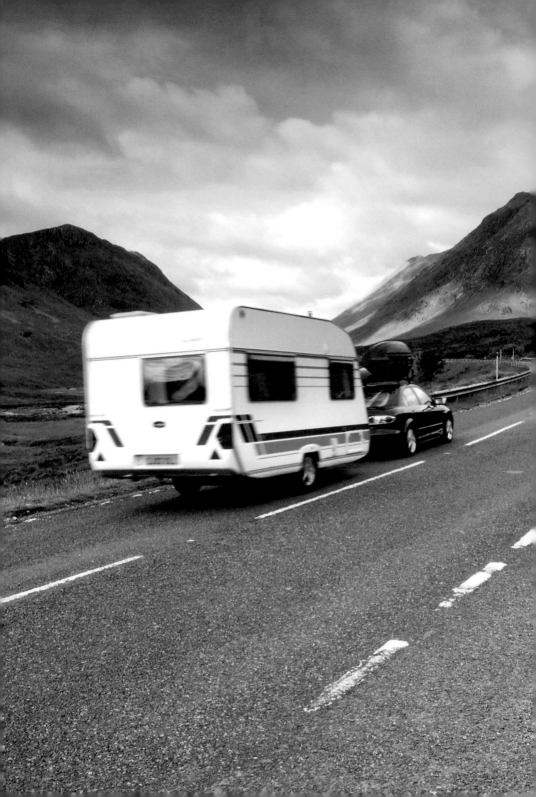

← Conventional touring caravans offer great comfort, and smaller ones can be towed by standard family cars.

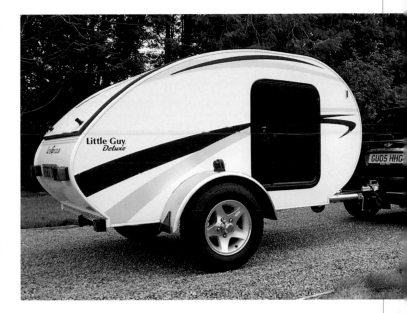

→ Teardrops look great and are easy to store and tow. You will bang your head. A lot.

Teardrop caravan

The name 'teardrop' comes from the distinctive shape of these retro-inspired travel trailers. The standard design is to have a bed area accessed through a door on the side, with a lift-up tailgate that encloses cooking, storage and utilities. These can be home-built or bought finished. They are niche, but look great and offer a surprising level of comfort.

Lifestyle caravans

These are typically caravans that are smaller, stylish and lightly equipped. They are often purchased to facilitate a hobby, or simply because they look nice in the back garden as an outside spare bedroom. They're great for weekends and short breaks, but many are a little tight on space for extended touring

Classic caravans

Caravans have been mass-produced since the 1960s, and the basic form remains unchanged. As a result, they can be used like any other caravan. Classics often need ingenious remodelling to keep them serviceable as some spare parts can be an issue, but there is a vibrant scene and the best ones are worth strong money. Beware that headroom is often limited.

⬇ Style-focused tourers such as the Bigfoot look great, but aren't the best for longer tours.

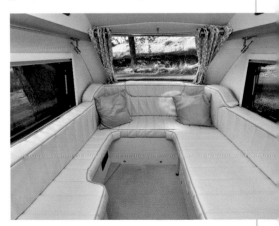

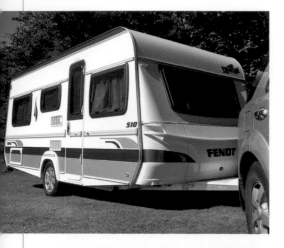

Touring caravan

This is what most people picture when they think of a caravan. Most are white boxes with a broadly uniform external appearance, equipment and running gear, regardless of size. The main differences are in body length and width, and the number of axles. Larger ones have two axles to spread the weight. These are the caravans you find at regular caravan dealerships.

← There is a caravan for every buyer. Newer, larger ones are plusher and have more storage, but smaller ones are easier to work with.

What is an awning?

An awning is a fabric extension of the living space. Caravans work perfectly well without one, but most do have at least one. They come in all shapes and sizes, ranging from the surprisingly affordable to eye-wateringly expensive.

The simplest form of awning is a fabric sun canopy attached to the caravan awning rail – an aluminium extrusion built into the side of every modern caravan. These are more popular with Continental tourers – the British caravanner tends towards something more weatherproof.

Porch awnings typically cover a proportion of the side of the van either side of the door, meaning you can store muddy boots outdoors without them filling up with water.

Porches fit a variety of caravans, regardless of size, which means they tend to be cheaper than full awnings, which need careful measurement to ensure a good fit. Full awnings essentially double the size of the accommodation, but bulk and weight mean that they only tend to get used when staying on site for longer periods.

Awnings range from a couple of hundred to several thousands pounds, depending on what exactly you need. Looking after them is important and you should apply the same rules to them as you would a tent: careful handling, keeping them clean and not putting them away damp are all essential if you want to maintain them.

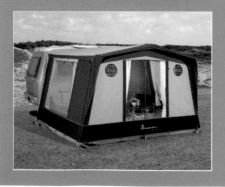

← A full awning can effectively double your on-site living space.

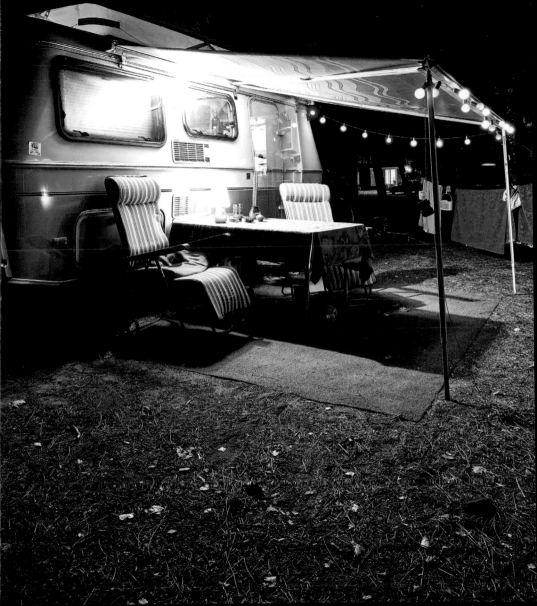

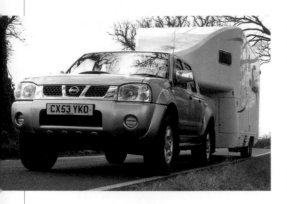

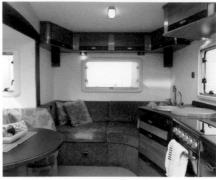

↑ Fifth-wheel units are rare and need a modified pick-up to tow them.

↑ The plus side of a fifth-wheel caravan is excellent on-site accomodation and lots of kit.

Fifth wheels

These caravans need a suitably equipped pick-up to tow them as they use a dedicated trailer attachment, the 'fifth wheel' in the pick-up bed. They are a bit niche, but typically offer pretty palatial on-site accommodation. The market is quite small for this type of unit, so they usually need to be sourced directly from the importer or manufacturer.

Travel trailer

This is really an American idea, and few travel trailers are found in the UK. They are large, and many are crudely screwed together, but often feature eye-catching specifications. They tend to be placed on site for long periods – years, rather than months – due to difficulties moving them around. The Airstream is one of the few built for European use.

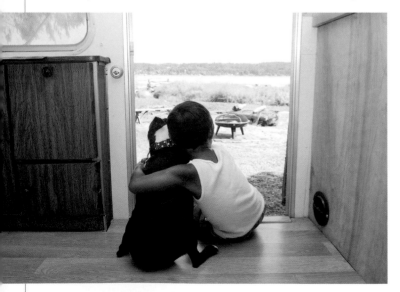

← Smaller vans are easier to pull up in roadside picnic areas to make impromptu stops.

Choosing a caravan

As to which of these will suit you best, it's hard, but not impossible, to say. Trailer tents, folding campers and teardrops are perhaps best considered as an easy upgrade for tent campers tired of lying on the floor. To take on a classic caravan, you really need to want to do the work that will inevitably follow, but they can be beautiful.

At the other end of the scale, travel trailers and fifth-wheel units are really for those with enough experience to know they are going to like them. In both cases, they are quite expensive to buy but hard to sell other than to specialists.

All of this means that for most people, standard touring caravans and appealing lifestyle vans are a great place to start. The more lifestyle caravans, such as the T@B

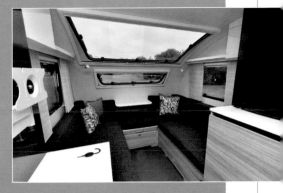

↑ The Adria Action is a small van, but uses the space smartly. The windows stop it feeling stuffy.

and the Swift Basecamp, are great for the first-timer, particularly if they aren't sure that caravans are for them. The standard touring caravans are where most will end up, though. There are loads to choose from, at a variety of layouts, prices and masses, meaning most people will find something that suits. The only way to know for sure is to go to have a look at some.

↓ The stylish baby Adria is proof that modern caravans don't have to look boring, or need an SUV to tow them.

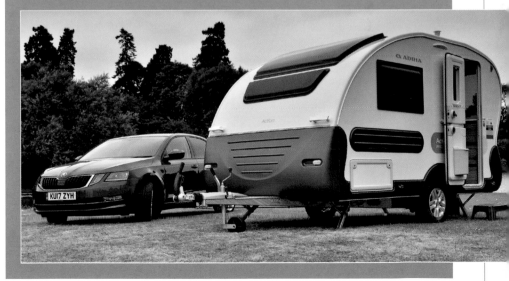

What is a tow car?

To move a caravan, you need a vehicle with a tow bar. What size and type of vehicle this should be depends entirely on what you are towing.

Small family cars are perfectly adequate if you are eyeing up a folding camper or small tourer. It's only when you get up into the bigger, heavier trailers that you need to start sizing up to four-wheel drives and pick-up trucks.

There are some vehicle types that cannot tow. Ones that have not been homologated for towing are a no-no, although you may still find tow bars for them. Usually, these are used for attaching bike racks and the like. Things like small sports cars and smaller hybrid-electric cars are in this category.

Generally speaking, diesel-engined cars are better for towing, mainly because they deliver their power without having to work as hard, so the engine is less stressed and less fuel is burned. Typically, a diesel car is heavier, too, which means it is easier to get a good car–trailer mass match – more on this later. Larger-engined or turbo-charged petrol cars make excellent tow cars, but fuel economy is often disappointing.

⬇ Older caravans such as the Bailey Ranger tend to be lighter and can be towed by smallish cars. They are great starter vans.

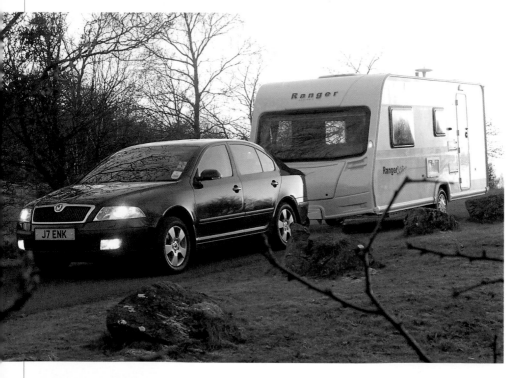

→ Larger, heavy vans such as the short-lived Stealth need large, powerful cars to tow them safely.

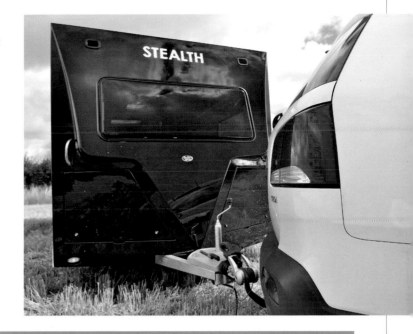

Driving licences

The size of trailer you can legally tow is dictated by two things: your driving licence and your tow car. On the back of your driving licence, the categories of vehicle you can drive are displayed in a table. The one you are looking for is category B. If you passed your driving test prior to 1997, you will have B+E categories already. That means you can tow pretty much any caravan behind any car.

Difficulties occur if you passed your test in 1997 or later, as outlined on page 37. Your options are far more limited. The maximum you can tow in this case is the combined gross mass of the tow car and caravan, which must be less than 3,500kg (3.44 tons) in total.

That sounds like quite a lot, until you remember that these calculations are done on the maximum mass of the car, not the kerb weight. That means something as ordinary as a Ford Mondeo 2.0-litre diesel tips the scales at nearly 2,200kg (2.17 tons), leaving you just 1,300kg (1.28 tons) for your caravan, which, as you will come to see, is quite a restriction.

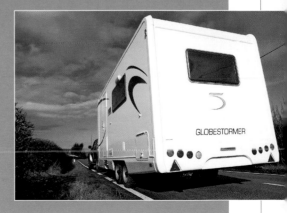

Laws and physics

We can't go much further without covering some of the technical boring stuff – namely, towing weights and manufacturer's specifications.

First, you need to work out whether your prospective combination of car and caravan is a legal match. For that you need four pieces of information:

W = Car kerb weight
X = 85 per cent of car kerb weight
Y = Maximum towing limit of the car
Z = Maximum technical permissible laden mass (MTPLM) of caravan

- Your car and caravan are a legal match if Z is equal to or less than Y.
- Your car and caravan are a recommended safe match if Z is equal to or less than X.

- Your car and caravan are an acceptable match if Z is between X and W.

To make this a little more manageable, let's use a couple of examples.

A car has a kerb weight (W) of 1,200kg (1.18 tons) and a maximum towing limit (Y) of 1,400kg (1.38 tons). This means that X is 1,020kg (1 ton). This mass – 1,020kg (1 ton) – now becomes the target MTPLM of any caravan we are looking at as it is a good match.

⬇ Check your car's chassis plate and use the handbook to decipher it.

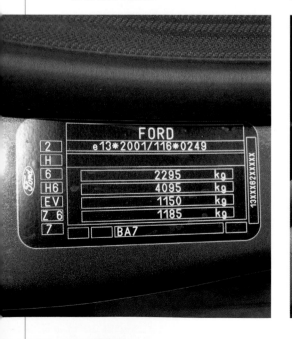

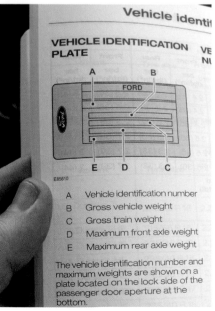

A   Vehicle identification number
B   Gross vehicle weight
C   Gross train weight
D   Maximum front axle weight
E   Maximum rear axle weight

The vehicle identification number and maximum weights are shown on a plate located on the lock side of the passenger door aperture at the bottom.

The 85 per cent 'rule'

You are likely to hear about the 85 per cent rule as soon as you start researching car and trailer masses. It is a useful rule of thumb, but it is important to remember that it is a guideline for novice tow-car drivers, rather than a law.

The idea is centred on the basic rule that it is better for the stability and comfort of a car and trailer combination to have a heavy car and a light trailer. This is entirely correct. The two main caravanning clubs, the National Caravan Council and others, settled on 85 per cent of the car's kerb weight being a sensible ratio to the maximum mass of the caravan.

The issue is that as time has worn on, cars have got lighter by a significant amount and caravans have been laden with more and more kit. That means in order to conform to the 85 per cent guideline, you need a large car for even fairly modest caravans. Factor in the restrictions placed by post-1997 driving licences and it is plainly harder than ever to hit this ratio.

If conforming to that ratio is proving impossible, exercise common sense. Go for the lightest caravan you are comfortable in, then transfer heavy items from the caravan to the car if practical. Avoid any match where the caravan equals or exceeds 100 per cent of the car's kerb weight. It may be legal, but you are reducing the margin for error and minimising your outfit's natural stability. In short, your risk of an accident is higher.

If your outfit is within the recommended limits, loaded carefully and driven sensibly, you will have every chance of a safe, stress-free journey.

To complete our example, let's say we are looking at two caravans to match with our car.

Caravan A has an MTPLM of 1,000kg (0.98 tons) and Caravan B has an MTPLM of 1,150kg (1.17 tons).

Using this information we can see that the MTPLM of Caravan A is slightly below our X mass so is a good match. The MTPLM of Caravan B is between our X and W figures, so it is at the heavy end of acceptable and may not be ideal for a novice.

Matches in which Z is higher than W, but lower than Y are legal, your personal driving licence permitting, but not recommended.

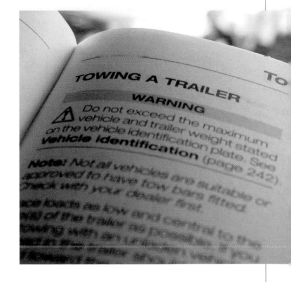

↑ Your car handbook will have information on best practice when towing. Read it.

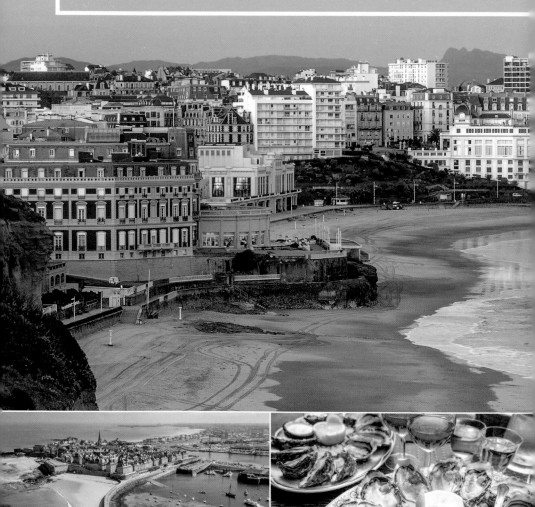

Van Life Inspiration
The French Atlantic Coast

While the Cote d'Azur gets all the attention, the vast and varied Atlantic coast of France is a vastly better van destination. The cool, wild Celtic coast of Bretagne in the north gives way to more pastoral landscapes as you head south around the Bay of Biscay. Stress-free, good value and culturally rich – it's a fabulous route to sample European touring.

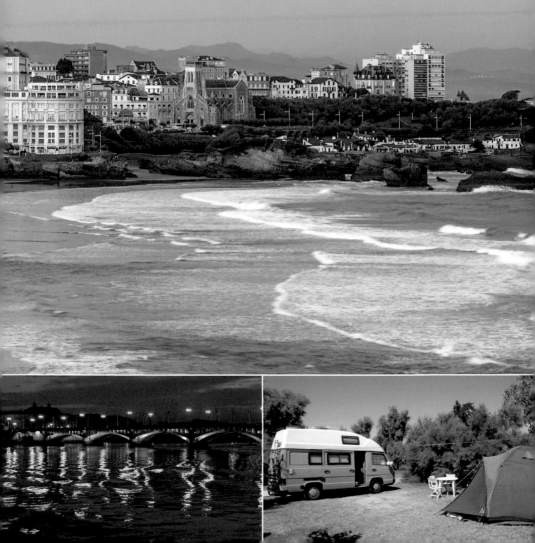

Time to buy

If you know the mass you are aiming for and you know how much you have to spend, you are pretty much ready to start shopping. Now you can think about what is going on inside the caravan, rather than outside or underneath it.

A big consideration is whether you want to build your bed from sofa cushions every night. This sounds like an easy decision, but if you choose a van with a fixed bed – one with a dedicated mattress – you are going to end up with a longer caravan, and unless you go for something very large, you'll have quite a small lounge. Many have quite snug washrooms, too.

Other configurations such as fixed bunks, large end washrooms and L-shaped lounge areas all introduce their own compromises. An entire book could be dedicated to the various quirks of

↓ Dealer sites will have a large selection of vans, both new and used.

caravan layouts, but this isn't that book. The only way to know what suits you is to don some comfortable shoes and go and look at some caravans. You'll quickly establish what you like and what you don't.

When you find features you like, make a note of them. It is vital to record the make, model and year of whichever caravan you are looking at. That way, if you want to scan the classifieds, you can focus your search a little more. It is no good just recording part of the detail either. Saying you liked a Swift Challenger Sport only narrows down your online searches a little – there could be 10 or 12 different layouts spread across five model years. Get as much information as you can.

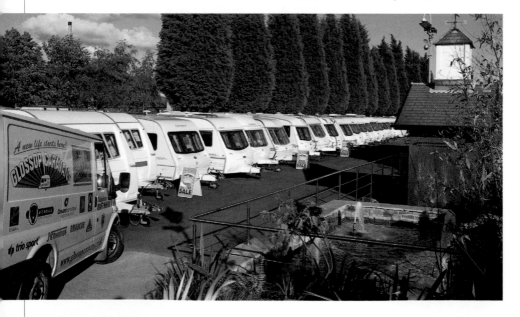

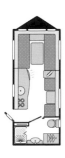 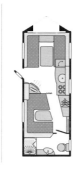 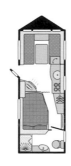 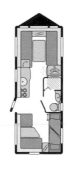 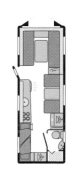

↑ One type of van can have loads of layout variations. Make note of the make, model and year of any that you like.

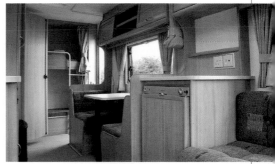

→ The only way to understand interior layouts is to go and see a few. You'll quickly get your head around the basics.

If you manage to find a layout you like, it's a good time to collar someone on the staff at a dealership forecourt for a chat. Many (but not all) sales people are knowledgeable and helpful, so if you say 'I like this but I want something lighter/ cheaper/smaller', they should be able to tell you your options. If they try to twist your arm Into buying the one in which you are sitting, despite what you've said, you've got the wrong sales person.

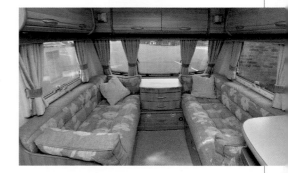

Shopping for starter caravans

When weighing up your first caravan purchase, you understandably might want to spend a little less than dealer prices to work out whether caravanning is for you. Dealers tend not to bother with caravans below around £5,000, although there are exceptions. If they do have that sort of stock, It is often marketed with minimal preparation on eBay or Gumtree, alongside privately marketed caravans. When buying cheaper caravans, it is vital

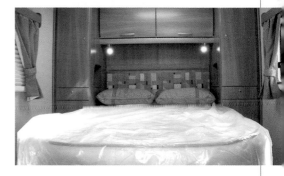

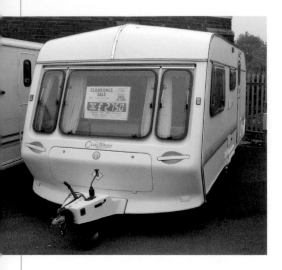

↑ Not all dealers sell more affordable vans. As a rule, the posher the dealer site, the less older stuff they will keep. Never hurts to ask though.

to put its condition ahead of any other considerations, other than whether you can legally tow it. It is definitely worth compromising on layout, preferred make or model or some other detail for an otherwise exceptional caravan. Spending less money means investing more time in researching the market.

Quite often, there is great value to be found at this end of the market. Caravans sold by owners are often bundled with expensive extras that are tricky to sell on separately. A new awning can cost anything from £250 to £4,000, depending on the make and model, but caravans sold privately often come with them thrown in. The same is true of security kit, motor movers, leisure batteries and all manner of other items. Dealers will commonly remove these from vans that are traded in or resell them as extras. Don't judge them, they are trying to make a living, but be aware that you can often get a better deal privately.

If you are buying privately, there are a number of caveats about handing over large amounts of money for high-ticket items and a few things you should do to keep yourself away from potentials scammers. Apologies if you have heard them before.

Caveat emptor means 'let the buyer beware' and that is the brief legal term that covers the level of protection you get as a private buyer. Virtually none. It's your responsibility to check that the caravan is in the condition you think it is and that it is the seller's vehicle to sell.

The seller must give an accurate description, but it can be hard to prove it if they pulled the wool over your eyes – so keep copies of the original advert. If the seller describes the caravan over the phone, ask for confirmation details by email.

Typical advice about buying a used car says you should insist on viewing it at the vendor's house to prove they don't mind you seeing where they live. However, this is not always practical with a caravan – many are kept at storage yards. Seeing the caravan at a proper storage unit isn't a problem. Seeing one in a farmer's field is less good. Use your instinct and take a friend for a bit of moral support, and for safety.

If you like the look of the caravan and the deal, then the last check you can make is to use a paid-for service called the Central Registration & Identification Scheme (CriS), which weeds out caravans with hidden histories. This service uses the caravan's chassis number – known as a CRiS number or Vehicle Identification Number (VIN) – to see if it has been reported stolen. It is £15 well spent. It is a voluntary registration scheme, however, so if the caravan has changed hands a few times, the registration details may not be completely up-to-date.

Common makes and models

The UK caravan market has traditionally been fairly loyal to UK-built products. This isn't just a bit of good, old-fashioned patriotism; UK caravans have their doors on the UK nearside because that is the side next to the kerb – the opposite side to caravans from elsewhere in Europe. The main names to look out for are Swift, Sterling, Bailey, Elddis, Coachman and Lunar. All are UK-built and still being produced. Alaria and Buccaneer are premium brands produced by Lunar and Elddis respectively. Adria are Slovenian-built caravans, but with plenty of UK-specific layouts, including doors on the correct side. Other brands, such as Hymer, Eriba and Knaus, are brought into the UK in smaller numbers. All are positioned at the mid to top end of the market.

In the second-hand market, there are a lot of makes that are no longer produced, but are still plentiful. The production of Abbey and Ace models was stopped in around 2008, but these were made by Swift Group and prices have remained stable. The Fleetwood name was retired by Adria in similar circumstances.

Avondale Caravans were made until about the same time, but the company no longer exists. Most major parts can still be sourced, but prices are depressed compared to those of contemporaries. Production of ABI Caravans stopped in 2001. Any of these makes need careful inspection due to their age, but they were well regarded at the time.

Beyond that, other caravans you will find for sale will be small-scale imports such as LMC or Hobby, low-volume coachbuilts from the likes of Carlight and Vanmaster, or other oddballs. They are not bad, but insurance issues and difficulty sourcing parts may well blight your enjoyment.

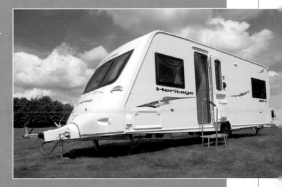

↑ The last of line Fleetwood models were nice to look at and had some interesting layouts.

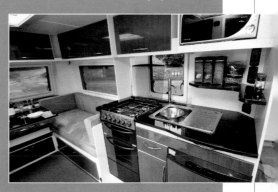

↑ Weird models such as Stealth and Eterniti are well equipped, but parts are impossible to find.

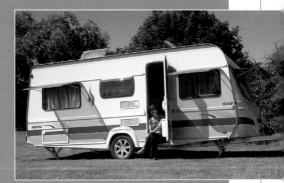

↑ Imports from manufacturers such as Fendt can be good value, but check you can get insurance.

Beyond the white box

The popular perception of a caravan is a big white box stuffed with floral furniture. That's wide of the mark these days, but for some potential suitors, the image is enough to put them off. All it takes is a few minutes' browsing the internet, though, to see that there are plenty of caravans on the market that are not scared to break the mould.

Eriba's Touring range of baby trailers has been around since the early 1960s, and despite constant product development, today's models still bear a striking resemblance to the originals. They are big on quirk, with elevating roofs and optional stripy sunshades, but even the bigger ones are fairly small. They were also built for pragmatic reasons; they are small and light, and that never goes completely out of fashion in the world of caravans.

⬇ Building your own unique camping trailer is perfectly possible with a basic workshop, help from the internet, and a lot of time.

What really kicked off the idea of a good-looking lifestyle-focused caravan was the Tabbert T@B. Launched in 2004, the idea of a small, sparsely equipped caravan with limited headroom didn't sound like a winner, but the fact that it remains in production, virtually unchanged, more than 14 years later is testament to a job well done. The range has developed and layouts have been modified but the basic shape is unmistakable and perfectly proportioned. They cost as much as a regular caravan, but scarcity means they are fairly resistant to depreciation. You won't find a cheap

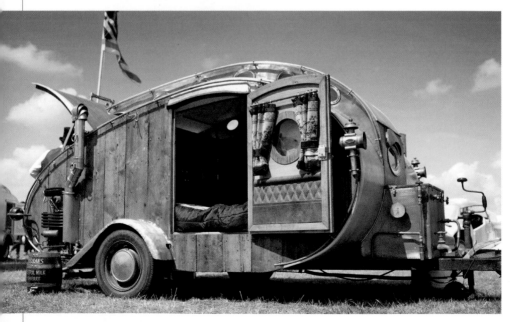

one, but you'll never lose money, either.

Another long-stayer is the Adria Action, which has been on the market in some form for a decade or so. Over the years, the wild blue windows and teardrop front window have gradually been toned down, but it has retained bold body mouldings and unique layouts that set it apart. The option of a fixed bed with a huge storage area underneath is a very clever bit of packaging for a caravan that is under 15ft (4.5m) long.

The newest entrant to this particular market is perhaps the one that makes the fewest compromises in terms of kit and comfort. The Swift Basecamp is, by most measures, a normal caravan, but it doesn't look like one. Billed as 'crossover camping vehicles', they are short and festooned in

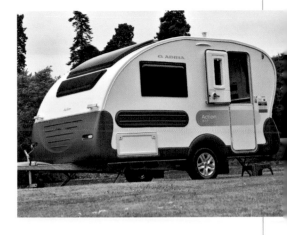

⬆ The long-lived Adria Action adds a degree of plush practicality to the traditonal teardrop trailer.

⬇ The Dub Box apes the classic lines of the original VW Transporter to ensure users stand out from the caravan crowd.

bold exterior colours and mouldings, meaning they look like nothing else you'll find on the forecourt. Despite their appearance, though, you miss out on few of the comforts you expect to find in a big white box.

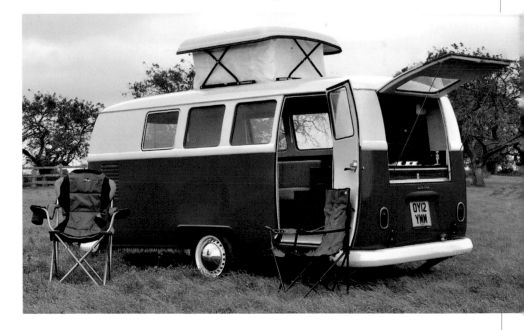

Tempting teardrops

Perhaps the prettiest end of the caravan market is the smallest end, where the tiny teardrop tourers reside.

The idea of the compact travel trailer came from magazine articles in *Practical Motorist* (UK) and *Mechanix Illustrated* (USA), which featured sets of instructions on how DIYers could make their own using basic techniques and simple materials. Each teardrop built this way was different, made to suit the builder and the materials they had to hand. The idea is especially popular in the USA and Australia, but these cute units are rapidly gaining popularity in the UK.

The teardrop name comes from the distinctive body shape that these compact caravans typically have in profile – humped at

⬇ Tiny teardrop models offer a very easy life on the road but less so on site. Think of it as a bed on wheels rather than a mobile home.

the front and sloping gently to the rear. They are small, too – typically, they stand little more than 4.9ft (1.5m) high and 13ft (4m) long.

The classic teardrop layout has a double bed in the 'hump' at the front, with a lifting tailgate at the rear, which covers the kitchen. Storage tends to be distributed among the various nooks and crannies in the corners and shelves of the curved bodyshell. Access to the bed area is through a small side door. Basic ones have little in the way of equipment, but the best have mains power, fridges, lighting and all manner of little luxuries that you might not expect to see in such modest accommodation.

If you don't fancy doing it all yourself, you can buy plans for a self-build teardrop on eBay or Amazon for around £20. If that is a bit of a stretch for you practical skills, Fyne Boat Kits will sell you a kit of parts with instructions for less than £2,000.

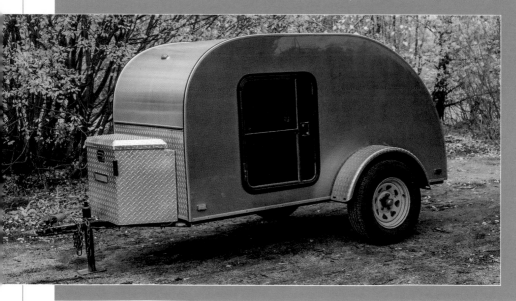

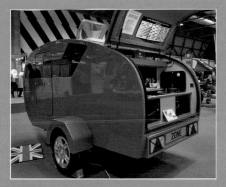

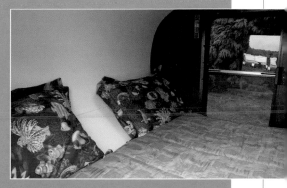

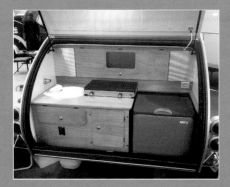

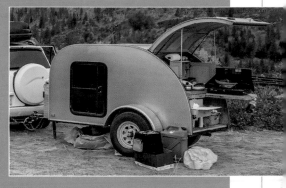

⬆ Typically, the kitchens are set at the rear of the trailer and covered by a tailgate. This keeps cooking smells away from the sleeping area.

⬆ In the right places, a teardrop can be more easily used for discreet overnight stops than a conventional caravan.

You don't need to do any of it yourself if you don't want. Companies such as Diddyvans will deliver you one of their Standard teardrops for less than £5,000, leaving you to accessorise and customise to your heart's content. Just add bunting. It's a lot easier than building one.

At the top end, companies such as Teardrop Trailers will build you a very high-quality teardrop with all mod cons, but a small caravan is just as much effort to make as a big one, so prices aren't as small as the caravan you are buying. Don't expect much change from £10,000.

If you want something a little bigger, the sharp-suited Go-Pod is bigger than a teardrop, and thanks to a campervan-style pop top, you can even stand up to get dressed. The layout is broadly similar to that of a traditional teardrop with a bit of 'boat' thrown in. The bed is at the front and the kitchen is at the back. The difference is that the whole lot is inside, accessed through a door at the back. The bed area is also a nice dinette by day. All this, but at a mass that means you don't need to worry about your driving licence and virtually anything can tow them.

Before you hit the road

Every time you use a caravan, you need to make some basic checks, but the first time you tow a new caravan, you should be especially vigilant. You don't take caravans for a test tow, so you'll only find out how it handles when you pick it up.

Don't take to the road without carrying out the basic requirements that ensure you stay legal. Towing a caravan you don't know needs concentration, so having to keep an eye out for police cars because you have a home-made number plate, no towing mirrors or something else obviously amiss with the van is not a good way to start. Make sure you've got an extra rear number plate, sticky pads and towing mirrors.

Towing mirrors can be tricky to fit, so practise before you go to collect the van. Unless you have a very narrow caravan, they are a legal requirement so that you get a proper view of the full length of both sides and behind the caravan. Good ones cost around £50.

Connect the towing electrics to your tow car to ensure all the lights work. It's common for caravan lights to stop working when they are laid up for a while. Typically, they can be got going by wiggling the bulbs or checking the electrical plug is not bunged up with dirt. A can of PlusGas or WD-40 is great for cleaning up crusty connections.

Tyres are a bit of a concern, too. You can visually check them *in situ*, but try to stop at a petrol station after a couple of miles to give them another check, ensure they are inflated and to look for evidence of any structural issues.

⬇ Smug people with big cars will tell you they don't need extension mirrors. Ignore them. They do.

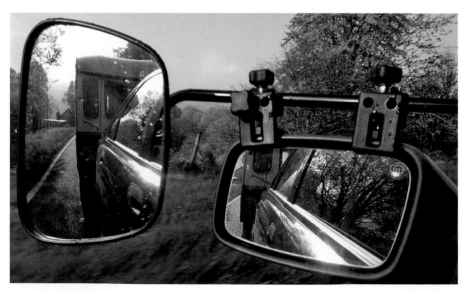

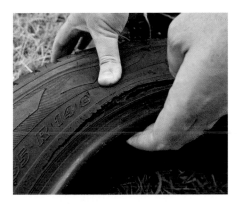

⬆ Have a good look at your tyres, every time you tow. Check the pressures and look for damage.

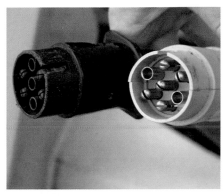

⬆ Check electrical connections and cables are clean and undamaged.

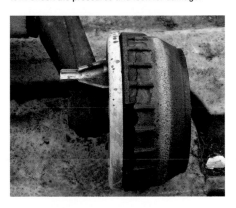

⬆ If the handbrake is left on, or badly adjusted, the brakes will heat up and seize. Expensive.

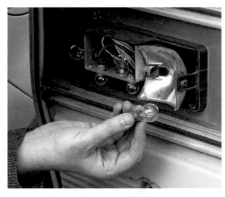

⬆ Caravan lights love to pack up for no reason. Check they work before leaving.

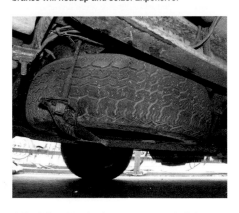

⬆ Don't forget to check your spare tyre is fit for use.

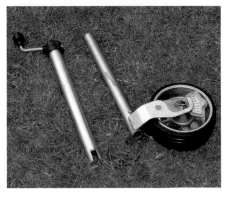

⬆ Ensure the jockey wheel stows and works correctly.

Case study

Humans	**Phil, Natalie and Harrison Owen, Tyler Lavery**
Dogs	**Bella, Atlas and Stanley**
Vehicle	**2008 Fleetwood Sonata Melody**

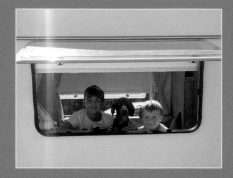

Phil and Natalie got the idea for buying a caravan after Nat's brother picked up their first tourer and immediately started spending every spare weekend whisking the kids off to sites in South Wales and Somerset.

'We realised they were having more fun than us and we wanted to do the same!' Nat said. 'We started looking at the small ads but it took a while. We looked at a lot of rubbish before we found our Fleetwood.'

The Owens' interest in owning a caravan wasn't just about holidays, however; Phil had a more pragmatic use for a prospective purchase in mind.

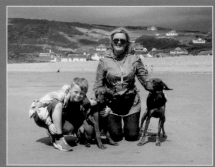

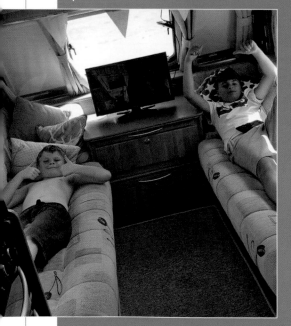

'I work away from home a lot,' he explained, 'spending weeks on end in the same hotel near to the power stations where I work. We started talking about getting a caravan, and it was all about having weekends away with the kids and the dogs. Then I started thinking that having my own space when working away would be a big upgrade on staying in hotels. I really wanted a fixed-bed but when we found the right van, it had a lounge front and back, with a kitchen in the middle. Everything else about it was

← Harrison (left) and Tyler (right) enjoy their time away in the van, spending their days running around with the dogs, cycling and playing football. They typically have the XBox on hand for evening-use though.

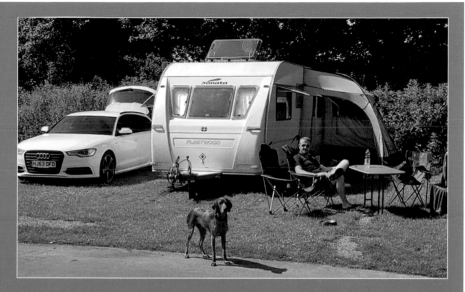

great though, so we put down a deposit and collected it a few days later.'

The Owens have a 2008 Fleetwood Sonata Melody and tow it with their Audi A6 Avant. Phil hadn't done a lot of towing before but wasn't fazed by it. The caravan saw a lot of use and the whole family got their skills up to scratch in double-quick time.

'It's great for the dogs, great for the kids and we love it too,' enthused Nat. 'When Phil comes back from a work trip, we jump in the van and spend a bit of time together. The kids take their bikes and Phil takes his barbecue so they are all lovely and quiet!'

It hasn't all been plain sailing, but the family has taken it in their stride. 'We had a problem with the fridge when we first got it, but that got sorted out pretty quickly,' said Phil. 'We also had some really rough weather one night. We all sat awake in the van with the wind howling, then there was a big crash from outside and we realised we had lost the awning. I dashed outside, grabbed all the scattered bits and threw them in the boot of

↑ The caravan serves a useful dual-purpose, providing comfortable long-term accommodation when Phil works away, and holiday lodgings when he comes home!

the car. The wind had calmed down by the morning so we repitched the awning, with a few running repairs here and there. The weather was lovely again the next day, but there were a lot of other people doing the same mending and patching up. It wasn't just us, so that made me feel less of a beginner!'

The other big beneficiaries of the new-found caravan life are the family's dogs, Bella, Stanley and Atlas. Natalie explains, 'Taking dogs on holiday can be a nightmare, even with a dog-friendly hotel or holiday park. Our lot are good as gold, but you are always nervous about leaving them in a hotel room or rented cottage, as it is not their space. If they chewed something or broke something – nightmare. In the van, they are relaxed, get plenty of company and – like the kids – if they are happy, me and Phil are happy too!'

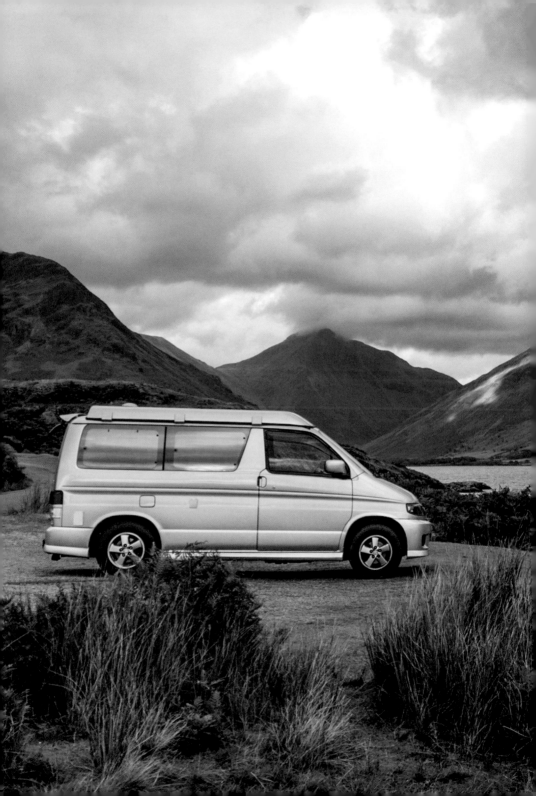

Chapter 5
The pragmatist's guide to van life

Search Instagram and it might appear that van life is all about doing yoga poses at sunset, or stopping halfway up a mountain for lunch with a view, but those things are the rewards. At least if you are into yoga. There is a lot of fun to be had spending your spare time on wheels but there are also a lot of practicalities to bear in mind. Getting a few basics squared off early on means you'll have more time to enjoy yourselves and there will be less chance of something unexpected derailing your adventure. Whichever form of van you choose, whether you go near or far or for months or hours, there arc plenty of practical skills that only come with knowledge or experience, or both.

Staying legal

Knowing the law is obviously very important if you want to stay on the right side of it. Some rules are obvious, but there are a few ways you can stray over the thin blue line without knowing you are doing it.

If you have a campervan or motorhome rather than a caravan, the rules are basically the same as for a car. Namely, you need to pay vehicle excise duty (road tax) and third-party insurance, and presuming that the vehicle is between three and 40 years old, you need an MOT too.

⬇ Wherever you travel, whether it's Brighton beach in the UK or this national park in Thailand, your van will need to be legal.

Bear in mind that if your vehicle would not be legally allowed on the road in the UK, it is not legal anywhere. That means you need to be up to date with road tax and have a valid MOT, wherever you are.

Although you will probably never get caught, the issue comes should you need your insurance or breakdown cover. Both are likely to be invalidated if the vehicle's paper trail is not complete.

That's all pretty simple but there are a few more things to consider. If you are

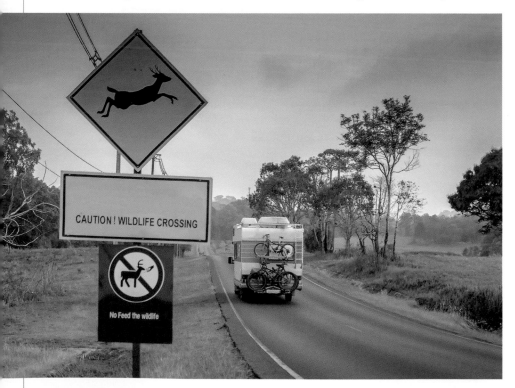

Do you need an international driving permit?

The IDP or international driving permit is a document that is used in conjunction with a regular full driving licence to prove that you are allowed to drive in countries that don't recognise a regular licence. Helpfully, it is a multilingual document that can help smooth the path when your language skills don't stretch quite far enough.

In Europe and countries nearby, a modern photocard licence will be fine and you don't need to worry about anything further. That said, the official advice from the AA is that if you are still persevering with a paper licence, you should get an IDP for countries as near home as Spain, Portugal and Italy to prevent problems with officials not accepting non-photographic ID.

As a general rule, if you are planning on driving outside of the EU, it is money well spent.

IDPs can be issued by certain Post Offices, but your local high street one may not know what you are talking about. For instance, there is one issuing office in the whole of Bristol, so check before you travel whether your chosen branch issues them. The Post Office website lets you search for branches that do.

In order to get one, you'll need a passport photo, signed on the back, your full UK licence and a completed application form. At the time of writing, the cost was £5.50. The IDP needs to be renewed every 12 months.

stopped by a police officer in another country, you will be expected to produce certain documents on demand:

■ Passport
■ Visa (if required)
■ Driving licence
■ International driving permit (only for countries needing it)
■ Your vehicle's registration document (V5C)
■ Your motor insurance certificate

The easy ones are passports for you and those travelling with you. For simplicity, keep details of any required visas to hand, too, as rummaging through your paperwork while a foreign police officer taps his or her fingers on the roof is about as much fun as it sounds.

Driving licences are a must, but since

they were switched to the photocard style, you have to renew them every ten years, unlike paper ones, which lasted from the date of issue until your 70th birthday. Ensure yours is valid for the duration of your trip. For certain destinations, you may need extra paperwork in the form of an international driving permit (see box).

A common question asked by officials when stopping a vehicle or making an enquiry is 'Is this your vehicle?' If the answer is anything other than a straight 'yes', you can expect more questions. The best way to demonstrate ownership is to produce your V5C registration certificate, which is the document you should have received when you registered the vehicle. Modern ones are presented in A5 size with a red cover, which clearly shows the details of the registered keeper and the registration mark. If for some reason you

MOT rule changes

The rules on MOT testing in the UK changed in 2018. There were some material changes to how the test is done and what is and is not allowed, but that's not the interesting bit. The thing to bear in mind is that vehicles that are 40 years old from the day they were registered are no longer required to have an annual MOT test. For the purposes of living in a van, that is one less thing to worry about, but as the driver, you are responsible for ensuring your vehicle is roadworthy. So, regardless of whether the van or tow car needs an MOT certificate, it needs to be roadworthy. Without the mandatory annual check-up, it is either up to you and your spanners to keep on top of the maintenance, or you and your wallet to pay someone to do it. Either way, as the driver, the responsibility is yours.

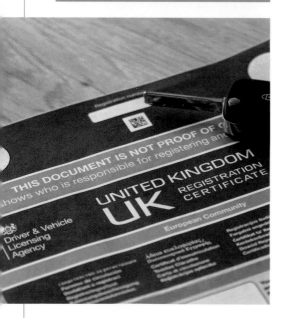

are not the registered keeper of the vehicle and they are not travelling with you, you need to demonstrate that you have the vehicle with their permission. For this you need to get a VE103B 'vehicle on hire' certificate. Typically, these cost under £10 and details on how to obtain one are on the DVLA website.

Your motor insurance certificate is another must-have. You must be able to produce proof that the vehicle is insured, but it is actually a useful document to familiarise yourself with anyway. It lists the countries that you are insured in, so if you are pondering a border crossing, you can quickly scan the paperwork to check that you are covered. It will also include details of whether you are covered to drive other vehicles, in case the need arises.

All of the above is perfectly fine if you are planning to be out of the UK for 12 months or less. If you are planning an extended stay abroad, however, you should get your MOT done fairly soon before you leave to give yourself maximum flexibility. You then have until the renewal date to get back.

More than 12 months away

If you intend to leave the UK for more than 12 months, there are some vehicle admin issues to consider before you start your extended adventure. If you are planning 12 months continuously outside of Blighty, you need to re-register the vehicle to the country you are heading to.

To do that, you need to get hold of your vehicle logbook (the V5C form). Fill out the section on the second page relating to permanent export of a vehicle, then begin the process of making your van legal in the country in which you plan to register it. Each country has different rules, but the basics for EU countries are as follows:

- Register the car with the relevant authorities
- Change the number plate
- Show proof of ownership and that you have the relevant roadworthiness certificate
- Pay registration, road tax and insurance for the new country

If you are planning on staying permanently outside the UK, that is all fine, but if you are living your best van life and freewheeling across the world, you won't be visiting just one specific country, and that leaves you with an issue: you won't be in the UK, but you won't specifically be anywhere else either, so re-registering is not feasible.

In this case, the simple solution is to factor in a return trip to the UK some time before the MOT expires. This gives you a chance to get a new test certificate and then bid farewell to the rain for another year. If your MOT lapses when you are outside the UK, you have no alternative other than to get it back to the UK for an MOT. You cannot get an MOT test certificate anywhere other than the UK and Northern Ireland.

Incidentally, there is an exception for lapsed MOTs, which is that you can legally drive a vehicle that is taxed and insured to a booked appointment at an MOT test centre. Internet forums are full of people saying they drove back from Budapest or Soweto to attend a booked test in Dover, so technically they were covered. Nobody seems to want to give a definitive ruling on the legality of this, and you might get away with it, but it is plainly outside the spirit of the rules and should you need to call on your insurance policy or breakdown service, you may well find yourself significantly disadvantaged. Don't risk it.

Van life myths

You can register a car/van with a SORN if it is not in the UK

You absolutely cannot do this just because you are not on the road in the UK. SORN stands for Statutory Off Road Notification and means you don't have to pay vehicle excise duty (road tax). If it is parked up somewhere and not in use, that is OK. If it is not on the road in the UK, but is on the road elsewhere, that is not OK. If it isn't legal at home, it isn't legal wherever you are.

You can get your car/van MOTed in Gibraltar

Not true. You must return UK-registered vehicles to the UK mainland for an MOT. Only vehicles registered in Gibraltar can be MOTed there.

Non-MOTed vehicles can legally be driven to a booked appointment at a test centre

Well, yes, but this arrangement is in place to allow you to drive to your local MOT centre, rather than to cross a continent or multiple countries to get to a UK garage. Legality on this is sketchy and insurance companies don't need much of an excuse to make life difficult. Inadvisable.

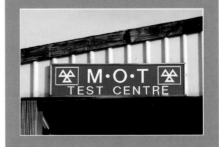

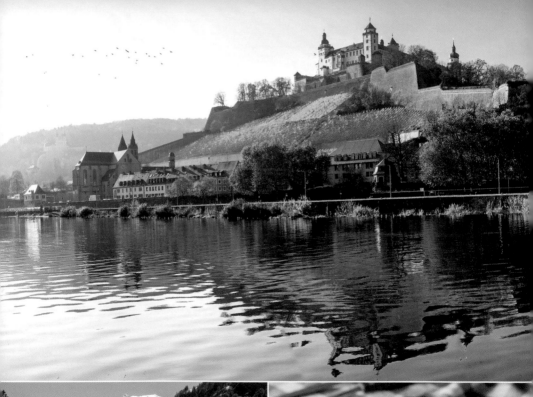

Van Life Inspiration
The Romantic Road, Germany

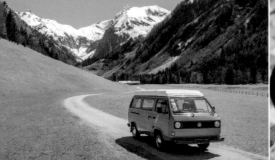

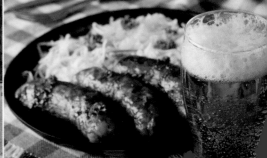

The Romantische Straße is a 220-mile route between Würzburg and Füssen that slips past the finest medieval castles and towns on the planet. Some of the basic route is authentically old, but much of it was enshrined by marketeers in the 1950s trying to tempt tourists to post-war Germany. It worked!

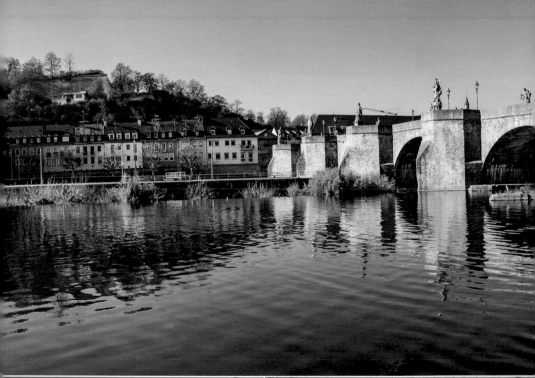

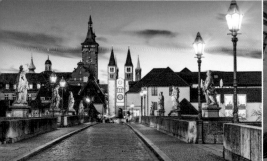

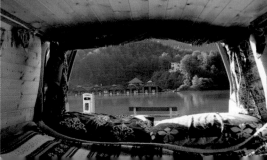

How to live a happy van life

It is hard to be definitive about what staying happy means as, obviously, it is highly subjective. For every person who likes to climb to the top of mountain, there are plenty more who like to sit quietly and read a book, or go tumbling into town on a push bike in search of local folk, food and fun. Whichever feels more like your van life, there are a few things to bear in mind.

Get along with your companions

Even the biggest van is a relatively confined space, so it is easy for cabin fever to creep up on you. If there is more than one of you travelling, it's very easy for even best friends or partners to start getting niggly with each other, too. Keeping your mood on an even keel is a huge part of enjoying the adventure.

The enemy of harmony when travelling with someone else is not talking about how they are getting up your nose. The most successful travelling companions are not afraid to disagree with each other. You don't want to be rowing all the time, but a sulky half-an-hour after a difficult discussion about snoring, bathroom habits or some other kitchen-sink drama is preferable to a full-on screaming match if things are allowed to build up and up. Before a wheel is turned, start off with a few ground rules or expectations and keep talking about them. As you travel, some will be forgotten and others will be firmed up but the dialogue is vital if you are going to enjoy your exploration.

The very nature of a van is that the space is confined so make sure you avoid spending too long cooped up inside. Long days of driving are very boring, you'll start to get uncomfortable, the radio will keep playing the same stuff and before long, you'll start to bang heads with your travel companion. More out of boredom than

anything else. At the first sign of that, find somewhere to stop and get away from the van. It could be a village, a field or a city, but stretching your legs and your mind with something new to think about is essential.

If you are travelling little and often, you should find there is enough stuff to keep everyone happy but sometimes you just need a little space and you should not fear that. Whether with a close friend or a partner, going for a wander alone is good. If nothing else, a couple of hours apart means you have something to talk about when you return. It doesn't have to be desperately exciting. A walk into town for a coffee can be more than enough to break any monotony. Exercise is great for clearing the mind and hitting the reset button. We aren't talking about running marathons. A brisk walk, cycle ride or some gentle yoga stretches on the bed can do wonders for your state of mind.

If you and your travelling partner have divergent views on what constitutes fun, don't be afraid to split up for the day either. Do day trips or attractions alone to ensure you don't feel you are subjecting your companion to a load of things they aren't interested in. If you know they are bored, you won't enjoy your visit as much. Get comfortable with the idea of not living in each other's pocket and it will benefit everyone.

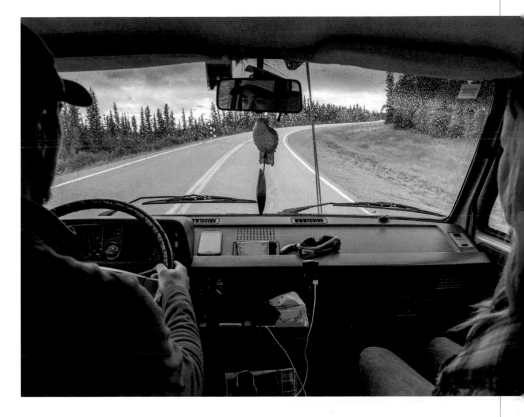

For couples travelling together, financial pressures are generally shared or at least managed and made someone's responsibility before you get in the van, so those arrangements tend to continue. If you are travelling with a friend, however, you should establish the rules over the financial arrangements early on. Standard arrangements are a straight 50/50 split on costs, or paying into a kitty, and documenting the outgoings as you go.

Also ensure you are clear on what happens if your van breaks. If the van is jointly owned by a couple, it's easy. If one person owns the van and the other is a guest, ensure that everyone is happy with where the costs lie. For example, the repair costs logically sit with the owner, but should

↑ Two people in a confined space is a recipe for conflict if you aren't careful. Keep talking to avoid any build up of tension or irritation.

the guest contribute, and what about hotel bills if you're grounded? Talk about this stuff ahead of time to ensure you don't end up making a stressful time even more stressy.

However you split things up, make sure that everyone understands how the money is being managed and that everyone is happy. Money is one thing that can bring even the closest friends to loggerheads if not handled sensible. If one of you wants to spend and the other insists on the most economical approach all the time, that is another great reason to make sure you spend some time apart on tour.

Suit yourself

A lot of people plan their free time when away from home around the expectations of people it has nothing to do with. For example, you might fancy a trip to Tuscany because of the pretty scenery and great food, but a lot of travellers feel some sort of perverse pressure to visit the region, just because they are in the country. If you want to go to Florence, go, but if walking around a city looking at old buildings and paintings isn't what suits you, don't do it. Do, however, make sure you talk to your travel companion(s) and ensure everybody gets a say in where you go, within reason.

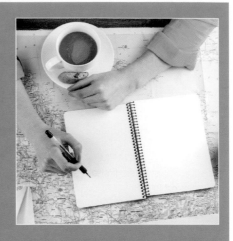

↑ Plan your trip in advance but make sure group decisions are made collectively.

Take your time

For shorter breaks, up to a month in duration, there can be a temptation to overcrowd the itinerary. When you are sitting at home with a map spread out on the floor with entire countries in front of you, it is tempting to pull together a hitlist of towns and attractions and insist on banging them all off during the trip. Such itineraries are fine, but they aren't for everyone.

Likewise, setting off with no plans at all can be exciting, but it can also be stressful for people who are planners by nature. The best solution is something between the two. Have a few solid touch points – places you plan to be in on certain days or weeks – and then fill in the gaps between. Fixed travel plans are a great example of such touch points. If you have a return ferry booked, you know where you need to be on that particular day. If there is a market day in a town, friends you are planning to catch up with or some other plan afoot,

pencil things in, and then let what you find along the way fill the gaps.

Not stressing about being in a particular place on a particular day is a key tenet of van life. The whole point of having a van is that you can suit yourself to a far greater extent than you could if you were renting an apartment, villa or hotel room. If you don't like a place as much as you expected to, move on. If a place that looked humdrum on the map and was ignored by the guidebooks turns out to be your dream destination, stay as long as you need.

To a freewheeling van life veteran, even writing this stuff down feels a bit unnecessary, but for people taking time out of their normal work life, bounded by schedules, meetings or maybe hectic social schedules, the thought of unplanned travel can be utterly petrifying. Don't tie yourself to a rigid plan, but plan enough so that you don't end up stranded 250 miles (400km) from the ferry terminal as they are raising the loading ramp.

Keeping yourself healthy

Keeping yourself healthy when rolling around at your own pace with no particular place to go does at least mean your stress levels will be easily kept in check.

First aid and other health essentials

The basics of keeping yourself healthy are broadly the same whether you are in a van or at home, but basic first-aid skills and a well-stocked kit are a must have. Basic first aid kits start from less than a fiver for a lightweight, single-person kit heading to £50 plus for the plusher, better-equipped packs, but the brutal truth is that without training, it might count for nothing. Basic first aid courses cost from around £50 but if you are employed, ask at work. If you are prepared to become an office first aider, your employer may foot the bill.

The main thing to supplement your kit with is any regular medications you need and you must know how to get replenishments when you are on extended tours. Repeat prescriptions will be issued in advance by your GP for lengths of time up to three months away, maybe more depending on the nature of them. Speak to your GP before you go to find out how you keep your drugs going if you are heading away for longer.

The ease with which we all traverse the world these days means folks are less clued up on what vaccinations and jabs they should be having before travelling. If heading out for an extended tour, as well as visiting your GP to ensure you are basically fit and well to travel, tell them where you are planning to point your van and they will update you on which vaccines you might need. While the combined diphtheria, polio and tetanus booster is free, along with typhoid, hepatitis A and cholera, all others must be paid for. With private jabs costing around £50 a go, you might need to start saving. The NHS Fit for Travel website lets you research your destinations before you go to see what you need to get. (https://www.fitfortravel.nhs.uk/destinations.aspx)

⬇ Taking simple precautions, especially with clean water and food prep, will help keep you well.

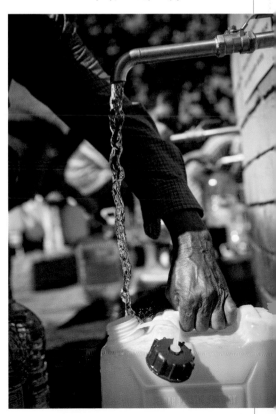

Mosquitoes, bugs and biters

Anyone who travels in hotter climes will have a plan for avoiding mosquito bites, and if you are lucky, some of them might actually work. Creams, potions and lotions too numerous to list here are on the market to repel biting insects but for every person who won't buy anything else, there is someone who will tell you nothing works. Science suggests Deet and oil of lemon eucalyptus work, but they will make you smell funny too.

The best advice with repellents is to experiment. Different things do work for different people, but always look at what you can buy locally. If the local pharmacist is well-stocked with a particular type of repellent, there is a reasonable chance it is effective on the native bugs.

Keeping flying bugs out of your van entirely is not realistic if you are touring somewhere with a lot of them, but you can certainly mitigate the numbers. Most motorhomes and caravans are equipped with flyscreen blinds which will offer some protection, so use those. Typically they aren't fitted on motorhome cab windows, so keep those closed and stick with the habitation windows.

If you are really struggling, then there is no reason you can't rig up a mosquito net in your van. In case you are not familiar, these are a fine mesh which is rigged up around a bed to keep bugs out. It's not 100%, but it is cheap, simple and silent.

We mention silence because many of the more 'active' solutions to bugs involve something you don't really want in your van. An ultra-violet zapper will wake you each time a bug is tempted to the light so is useless in a confined space. And citronella candles or burning solutions are a seriously bad idea in a vehicle full of timber and man-made fibres. Please don't leave things burning in the van while you sleep. A bite is better than a burn.

Other things to bear in mind is that biting bugs tend to like still water and still air conditions. If you are considered tasty by biting bugs, park the van away from ponds and lakes, and if at all possible, go for the most exposed pitch you can. A breeze is no friend of flying bugs and you will find numbers reduced if there is a squall. Seek out a little moving air if you can to make things more comfortable.

Finally, if you are in a place with loads of bugs, it is often easier to live with the bites than obsess over the bugs. Take antihistamines to reduce the swelling and skin irritation, stay cool but covered in light-coloured, loose-fitting clothing when in bed or walking about and definitely don't scratch those bites.

To cope with ailments when you are away, you should carry the basic medications that you know you are likely to need. Lemsip or cold remedies, over-the-counter painkillers, antacids, diarrhoea medications, antiseptic creams and other basics should always be in stock so you can administer basic care to yourself. Any symptoms that linger should be referred to the experts, however. For minor ailments, visiting a pharmacy avoids the hassle of finding and getting in to see a doctor.

For anything more serious, however, the pharmacist will be able to point you in the direction of a doctor or the local hospital. If not, a quick search on your smartphone will dig up what you need to get your sickness solved.

If you are nursing an ongoing condition, you owe it to yourself and any travelling companions to find out where the nearest medical facilities are and how to raise the alarm if anything happens. If you have medications for asthma, severe allergies, seizures, diabetes or anything else that can seriously debilitate you, ensure the medications are obviously located. If you feel an attack or episode is likely, wearing a medical ID bracelet is an excellent idea to improve your chances of getting the correct attention if you aren't in a position to explain.

The most common source of stomach issues when away in a van is likely to be from water. Bottled water minimises the risks of course, and across lots of northern Europe, you'll have no problems with drinking water from campsite taps anway. You want to be more wary the further you get from home and taking precautions using the van system makes sense anyway.

The enclosed water tanks in motorhomes are hard to effectively clean so drinking water straight from them if you haven't got a heavy-duty filter system, or haven't recently sterilised is a bad idea. Boiling water kills everything but you have a good 90-minute wait before you can enjoy a cold drink. Sterilising tablets will neutralise a lot of waterborne baddies but they taste rank, while 'taste' filters which are fitted as standard to many caravans and motorhomes will make the water taste better, but they don't kill viruses or bacteria.

A proper filter such as the General Ecology Nature Pure system will ensure what comes out of the tap is safe and palatable. These are designed to filter water from whatever source you can find while out and about, to turn it into something safely drinkable. It's an expensive system at just under £300 before fitting, but if it keeps you healthy, and reduces the amount of bottled water you need to lug about, it represents pretty good value. It also means that you should never find yourself without water you can trust, wherever you are.

EHIC

If you are travelling around EU countries you should definitely get hold of an EHIC for each traveller before you go. EHIC stands for European Health Insurance Card and was formerly known as the E111. These are supplied free but watch out for websites trying to charge you for them; ensure you apply directly through the government website at www.gov.uk/european-health-insurance-card.

Once you have one, the card entitles you to state healthcare in all EU countries, as well as Norway, Liechtenstein, Iceland and Sweden.

It doesn't necessarily mean you will get completely free care as happens in the UK, but it does ensure a minimum level of assistance and discounted access to services that might be subject to full private treatment rates otherwise.

The EHIC card should be considered the absolute minimum level of health protection for travelling abroad, and wherever you go, you should ensure you have adequate travel insurance in place.

TRAVEL INSURANCE

Travel insurance is traditionally sold in two flavours – single- and multi-trip – but insurers recognise that there is another

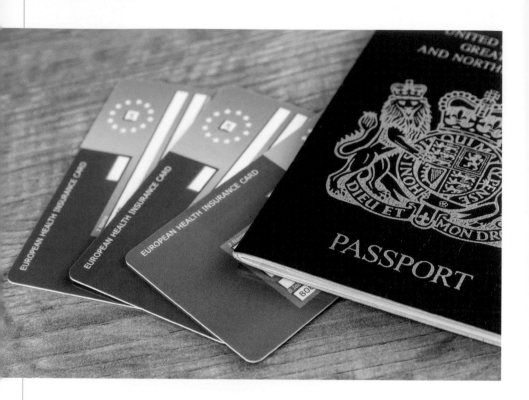

requirement that is now more commonly found: long-stay insurance. The main difference between these is the type of trips you are planning. A single-trip policy will typically cover an extended adventure of up to 100 days or more, depending on the policy, whereas multi-trip ones permit you to more than one adventure but of typically shorter durations, such as 60 days. The best long-trip policies will cover you being out of the country for 365 days. You need to consider which of these is likely to suit your needs.

Given the specialist nature of van travel, it is sensible to weigh up the value of specialist insurance. Long-term travel insurance options can be geared towards backpackers, for example, whose needs are different from those of van lifers. Additionally, cover for animals, children

⬆ The EHIC card is the bare minimum of travel insurance UK citizens should consider when touring around Europe.

and breakdown cover for the vehicle need to be considered, too.

Both major camping clubs in the UK – the Caravan and Motorhome Club and the Camping and Caravanning Club – offer policies that combine relevant travel and breakdown policies, for example, and they include specialist considerations such as repatriating a vehicle in the event of a breakdown or even providing a chauffeured return service if the main driver is incapacitated. Although these policies are only offered to club members, they will discuss the terms of the policy with you and quote for cover prior to membership, so you can see if it suits your needs.

Keeping your van healthy

For the majority of modern cars and vans, there is no problem getting things fixed if they go wrong outside the UK. If you are in Continental Europe, you may experience extended waiting times for parts that are right-hand-drive specific, but for most things, you'll have little to worry about.

If your van is a little out of the ordinary, it is a good idea to take a few spare parts with you. Older vans such as the Bedford CF are considered relics these days, while the tough LDV Pilot was simply never available in most of Europe. You will get bemused looks from mechanics if you roll up with one of these, so you need to give yourself the best chance of getting on the move quickly in the event of a breakdown.

The same is true for more modern machinery that has been imported from Japan. In the UK, the Mazda Bongo and Mitsubishi Delica are a relatively common sight due to the number of imports that have come over. The reason for their popularity in the UK but not elsewhere in Europe was at least in part due to the fact that they were right-hand drive. US-built RVs fall into the same category due to their relative scarcity on this side of the Atlantic.

It's impossible to predict the sort of things that might break, but carrying the basic service items should be considered a minimum. That way, at least you know that you can keep on top of the servicing and that breakdowns won't be due to poor maintenance. Carrying a set of oil and air filters, ancillary belts and front brake pads, for example, should be enough to get most mechanics started on an unfamiliar machine. If your vehicle has known foibles, such as air-cooled VWs with their fussiness over ignition components and spark plugs, pop a set of them in the back, too.

If you are towing a caravan around, there is generally a lot less to go wrong and the vast majority of the systems within the caravan are pretty uniform across Europe. That said, UK-built caravans are a rare sight in the rest of the world, so repairs to things like windows, body damage or heavy internal appliances, such as ovens or microwaves, may have to be patched up until you get back to the UK. Most modern tow cars present no problems to local garages, so unless you have something rare, you can rely on them to source most service items locally.

The majority of liveaboard equipment, such as fridges, cooking equipment or plumbing, is reliable and fairly standard in both caravans and motorhomes. It can therefore usually be fixed by competent caravan or motorhome workshops wherever you find yourself.

⬇ Breakdowns happen. Being prepared and having emergency cover on hand makes things bearable.

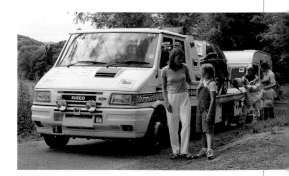

Case study

Humans **Steve and Jane Hogg**

Vehicle **2001 Hymer B584 and a 2007 Fleetwood Sonata Symphony**

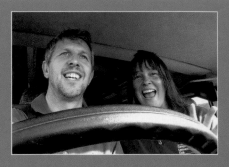

Steve Hogg and wife Jane have found the perfect way to blend a love of being outdoors with the need to make a living: they got a job working on a campsite.

'We've always loved being outside,' Steve explained. 'We've always loved camping, but then were given a 1972 Sprite and that was even better. We were hooked. We went away every chance we got. The problem was everything else. Work was getting in the way. I'd had 20 years working in an office and I thought, "Do I want to carry on doing this forever?"'

Inspiration struck soon after. Steve and Jane were sitting in their caravan, contemplating packing up after a weekend away, dreading work the next day when Steve glanced out of the window.

'I looked out and I saw this fella riding

⬇ When Steve and Jane take a break from their site warden jobs, they take their home with them and head off...in the van!

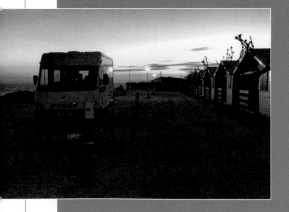

around on a little tractor. He was cutting grass, stopping and chatting to folk as he did and generally looking really happy. I thought to myself, "God Almighty, that's his job!"

I wanted to be that happy at work too, so we had a good talk about it and decided to take the plunge. We put together our application to be Holiday Site Assistants with the Camping and Caravanning Club and sent off the forms. We got a note back saying "Thanks, but no thanks," but we were on the list, so just had to wait until we were needed. No problem.

'We didn't have to wait long. We got a call out of the blue in April 2013 asking us if we wanted to work that season. That was it. Within a month, we'd rented the house out and sold every stick of furniture – well, everything we had. Storage was going to be really expensive, so we just got rid.'

'We had to buy a van, too. We sold the little Sprite, which was a bit too small to be our home, and we went looking on eBay. We found a 2007 Fleetwood Sonata Symphony at a price we could afford and a month after the call, we were pulling it on to the site. We left work at midday on Friday and by that same evening, we were behind the counter in reception, checking in the weekend visitors. We've never looked back.'

Steve says that it's important to think about a few things to make sure your time as a

Holiday Site Assistant is as great as his and Jane's. Steve says that they have come to realise a few things about the lifestyle, too.

'Obviously, you have got to want to do it, and you need to make sure you are happy with the money you earn and so on. Living full-time in a caravan isn't for everyone either, so it is important that you cancope with that.' 'We actually have a motorhome as well. We got a great deal on a 2001 Hymer B584 motorhome and, it sounds funny, but on our days off, we head out camping. You can sit on the site, outside with a glass of wine, but you always have an eye on what is going on. I call it the "warden twitch". You are constantly watching what is going on, looking at who is coming and going, even on your day off. People are always stopping for a chat, too. No problem at all, but it's not like you are ever fully off duty. So we found the perfect thing to do with a day or two off is to go camping! We jump in the van, and immediately, we are on holiday ourselves. We absolutely love it.'

The motorhome isn't just used for weekends away, however. The typical Club site season is from April to November and outside of these times, the Hymer comes in useful for getting further afield.

'It takes a week to wind the site down, to tidy up, do the final bits of maintenance and make sure the site is ready for the winter. Once it is done, we jump straight in the van, down to the Channel Tunnel and we are off. We have a book of aires and we make our way down to Spain. '

'We don't rush. We have plenty of time, so we set ourselves a limit of two hours behind the wheel a day. We stop in some lovely places. Sometimes one night, sometimes more, just driving from aire to aire. We do that for the whole winter, making sure we get back to the

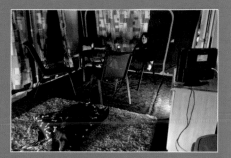

↑ Their van is set-up on site with an awning to give as much onsite comfort as possible

site a week or so before it opens to make sure everything is ready for when the gates open for another season.'

'For a lot of people, it is a job they think of as a retirement job but it's not for me. I'm 49 now, and I was mid-40s when we decided to do it. I started off as a Holiday Site Assistant and after a couple of years, moved on to become a Holiday Site Manager. Now I keep an eye on seven sites locally, but I am still based and work predominantly at Hayfield.'

↓ You can't be a fairweather camper if you work on a site. Make sure you get a van with excellent insulation and a good heater!

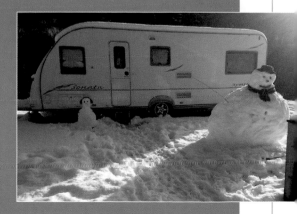

Staying safe

Staying safe when living in your van is straightforward but there are sensible precautions you can take to ensure you stay away from grief. While the perceived likelihood of issues may be high, life aboard a van is actually very safe indeed.

As a general rule, the less you rely on campsites and dedicated overnight or parking facilities, the more you need to take sensible precautions. The same goes for the places you go. The more exciting the destination, the savvier you need to be.

The main crimes that you are likely to encounter as a van dweller are theft, robbery and burglary. Happily, all are relatively rare. Simple definitions of the different crimes are pretty clear, and although there are different levels and qualifications, these demark the basic differences.

Theft involves taking another person's property without their consent and without

⬇ Caravans and motorhomes are valuable, desirable and a target for theft. Keep yours protected.

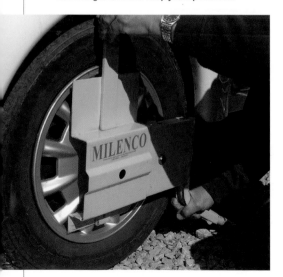

intending to return it. *Robbery* occurs when force is used or threatened against wa person in order to steal from them. *Burglary* is the act of entering a building as a trespasser with intent to commit other crimes such as theft, vandalism or assault. The first two can happen to any traveller at any time, but burglary is a specific threat to those in vans. We'll cover precautions concerning that later on.

Keeping thieves at bay

There is a lot of general advice for being a good tourist that is worth keeping in mind. It may seem a little basic, but it is never a bad idea to follow good advice, so it stands reiterating here.

Even the sleepiest, loveliest places can see careless tourists become victims of crime if simple precautions are not taken. Keep bags closed and keep your hands on them. Keep them close when outside cafes or restaurants and don't leave cameras and smartphones on tables while you are studying your maps and tourist books. The sort of folks who steal this stuff are depressingly well practised and your things can be snatched in a second. Vigilance is always the best defence.

When walking around, keep an eye on the areas you are walking around in. You are more likely to be a victim of a sneak theft such as a pickpocket attack in a busy area, but muggings and other personal robberies are more likely down quiet side-streets or cross roads. Don't avoid them –

that'll ruin your adventures, but be vigilant. What are popularly classed as the bad parts of town are often the most interesting. Stick to roads which have a few folks milling about, or some lights on. Keep your bags close and walk with a bit of purpose and confidence. Needless to say that dawdling down a poorly lit street and holding your smartphone up to look at a map is a bad idea.

Burglary

Your van is undoubtedly at the most risk when you are away from it. Motorhome parking areas around major cities are well known burglary hotspots. Criminals know a van is likely to be left unattended while the occupants are exploring the high-points of the local area. Plenty of time to hang about and when there is no-one around, pop open a window and have a rummage.

The standard advice here is to ensure there is nothing valuable on display through the windows which ensure your vagabond is guaranteed some booty to sell on. Small electricals are always a target due to high value and ease of trading on. You are likely to have your mobile phone and camera with you while exploring, so keep sat-navs, laptops and tablets tucked well out of sight. Ideally in an onboard safe.

That way, while you may have your van ransacked, your most expensive, precious or important items will be offered the best protection there is. If you don't have a safe, then your options are to keep things tucked in your sock drawer or to carry them with you as your get on with you touristing. Keep an eye on your bags though.

Other precautions worth investigating are additional locks for the van. For modern vans, a set of security deadlocks are easy to find and simple to fit. They don't make your van entirely thief-proof, but they will deter thieves after a quick smash and grab. Old-school steering wheel locks, pedal covers and a padlock and chain linking the cab doors all make the van less attractive to thieves.

Better than all these solutions is to park your van somewhere better. With caravans, leaving them on site and going into town by car is an option so not an issue. With a motorhome, renting push bikes, public transport or walking into town if close enough pretty much guarantee the safety of your van and its contents.

While attacks and robberies on motorcaravans in parking areas, aires and laybys are not unknown, they are certainly rare. Favouring official motorhome areas over laybys and motorway service areas certainly reduces the risk significantly, while opting for places with other vans gives a degree of additional peace of mind.

Other precautions

The main risk is simple anti-social behaviour – typically noise, car engines and rowdiness. The simplest solution to this is to move on to somewhere quieter. It is never good to remonstrate late at night with a group of rowdy folk in a language you likely don't understand. For that reason, keeping the van parked in a way that you can move on easily, ideally without external screen covers, means you can move off easily and quickly. If someone taps on the door to chat, experienced vanners suggest that answering through an open window or simply ignoring it is better advice than opening the door.

There have been plenty of reports over the years of 'gas attacks' on motorhomes and caravans while the owners sleep at rest areas. Reports are consistently that

If the worst happens

If you are unlucky enough to have to report a crime, having a bit of knowledge before it happens can help calm the inevitable anxiety that accompanies it.

All crimes should be reported and across most of the places you are likely to drive to from the UK, 112 is the phone number that gets you in touch with the authorities. Across the Americas, 911 is prominent, and in Oceania, a mixture of 999, 911 and 112 are used, depending on where you are.

When you head into countries that are a little off the beaten track, it is a good idea to note the numbers for the emergency services and pre-emptively look up the contact details for the embassy. It takes seconds to research and if you note it down and keep it to hand, it can save valuable frustrating minutes if problems occur.

Don't be surprised if you don't find an English-speaker on the other end of the phone, however, when you call emergency services. If you are lucky enough to have an English-speaking native to hand, getting them to make the call can save a lot of confusion. Try and convince them to hang around until the police arrive for the same reason. It can really help de-stress a situation.

Avoiding attention is not just about avoiding crime. Being a good tourist and a welcomed guest to an area is about displaying a little cultural sensitivity. You don't need to be accent perfect in the local language or conversant in local history, but you should be prepared to listen, watch and learn. That way, you'll get the most out of your visit and you are more likely to find doors into local life are opened just a little wider.

If you are heading to the beach, then

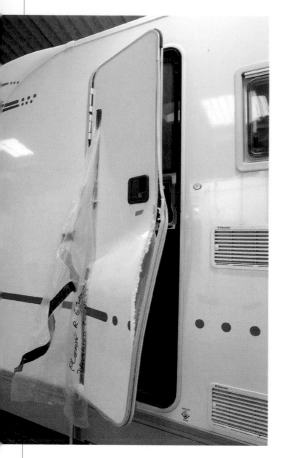

⬆ Burglary of a van can cause a lot of damage, so keep valuables out of sight and think carefully about where you park up.

the owners wake from a sleep with a headache and find they have been robbed. The popular explanation is that an ether-based anaesthetic gas has been used to knock the occupants out to facilitate the robbery. Opinions differ on whether or not this is actually feasible but for just over £100, you can equip your van with an ether-alarm, which goes off if knockout gas is detected. It's not expensive for the additional assurance it provides.

More tips for solo travellers

Vans are actually an excellent way to travel solo, and consequently it is not at all uncommon to find folks exploring on their own. After all, a van gives you as much social contact or solitude as you need. You can decide as you go along.

Much of the advice for solo travellers in a van is the same as any solo travel. Be vigilant, keep regular contact with at least one friend or relative at home so they know to be curious if they don't hear from you and keep key contact details close at hand, easily visible in a purse or wallet, or perhaps on the lockscreen of your phone, in case you have an accident and someone needs to be informed. We've mentioned issues regarding medication bracelets etc on page 139.

It is often the case that you end up crossing paths with folks doing similar journeys as you freewheel your way around. While everyone meets some people who they can't wait to get away from while away, if you encounter some like-minded travellers heading in a similar direction, swapping details is a great way of building a simple social network on the road which can prove very helpful if you get stuck, have a breakdown or simply fancy going into town for a beer with someone other than your dog for a change.

The advent of the smartphone is brilliant for managing this. If you do ever get stuck, whether it is a mechanical issue, health or you are simply unsure of where to go next, having the sum of all human knowledge available at the end of a web search is a huge boon.

Look after your phone, and ensure you have a top-up charger with you when out exploring. Used well, it can ensure you are never stuck, broke or lost for any longer than you need to be. Also ensure you familiarise yourself with the settings. Set it to backup your photos and contacts whenever it is on WiFi, so that if you lose or break it, you don't lose your memories and memorandums with the handset. Apple users can use iCloud for this, but Dropbox, Google and numerous other services offer similar clever set-ups which keep all your data safely backed up.

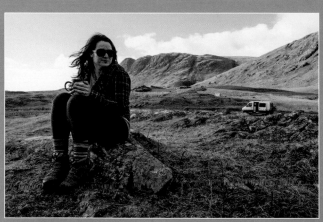

← A van is a great way to travel solo. There will always be people to talk to when you want to. And solitude when you don't.

swimwear is just about acceptable, but universally, walking around without a shirt, or in any form of revealing outerwear is basically frowned upon. Even in well explored places like France and Spain, it is considered poor form to parade around the town with too much skin on show. Keep shoulders covered and keep the legwear below the knee in western destinations.

If you head further east, then you want to tone things down further still to avoid coming across as ill-mannered or rude. Keep arms covered and long skirts or trousers are minimum requirements once you get towards Asia and into northern Africa. As a general rule, cover up more than you think, rather than less, and you'll likely be fine.

Aside from clothing considerations, there are other things which need thinking about on a place-by-place basis. While everyone carries at least one camera in the prosperous West, not everyone loves having a lens pointed at them. People are funny about photography around kids without permission, for understandable reasons but reactions of adults differ between cultures too. Some folks feel having a photo taken nabs a bit of their soul at the same time, so you can imagine why they don't like it. Don't take pictures without permission, and if you do ask and get given the nod to snap away in a shop or market, at least buy something modest as a thank you.

Be prepared to change your operating hours to suit the place you are visiting too. You won't be able to keep your normal eating times if dinner isn't served until the sun goes down where you are visiting. Watch and learn as you go and you will enjoy yourself all the more. Fighting the local norms will make you anxious.

On a potentially more serious note, keep an eye on local sensitivities. Gestures and actions which are harmless at home can cause unwitting offence in other cultures. Lean hard on good guidebooks to see what is acceptable and watch what others are doing. Don't think that ignorance of local customs will exempt you from local outrage. Eating on the street during Ramadan or disregarding the quiet days of the Hindu calendar can cause great upset and even see the police involved.

For solo travellers, there are more nuanced considerations, particularly for solo female travellers. All the things discussed previously apply, but extra attention is often paid to those travelling alone. For the most part, it is good-natured, occasionally intrusive calls to come and look at stores, stalls and restaurants. While it's great to get a flavour of the local folks and favours, sometimes, you want to explore at your own pace and bat away the attention.

A polite, firm refusal is generally enough to deter all but the most determined restaurateur or vendor. It is important to appear confident and comfortable (whether or not it is how you feel!) to enjoy your exploration on your own terms.

There a few practical accessories which can help diffuse attention too. A pair of sunglasses are considered by many to be a first-class deterrent to unwanted attention, minimising the chance of unintentional eye-contact when taking in your surroundings. When sat outside a Casablanca cafe, match the shades with a book or magazine to ensure you look like you need no assistance to enjoy your day. When you fancy a chat, pop them in your pocket.

Packing the right kit

The great thing about a van is that it has a load of space. People who go backpacking must fit everything in a nylon backpack, but you may well have a three-ton Transit to fill with gear, so you can lob everything in the back, right? Not right. Not even close.

When it comes to packing, enough is as good as a feast. You are much better off taking a few good-quality essentials with you, rather than packing absolutely everything you own. While you may have a generous payload to populate, it soon gets eaten away with profligate packing. You need to be utterly ruthless. And if you have space, you can pop a couple of nice bits in at the end.

⬇ There is a fine line between packing everything and slumming it. Think before you pack to ensure you tour with the right level of comfort.

We can't give a fully comprehensive inventory of things to pack, but the following is useful general advice:

Clothing

How much clothing you take is really a question of how frequently you want to visit a laundrette. After all, if you pack neatly, dirty washing and clean washing take up the same amount of space so if it all fits at the start, it will fit all the time.

Obviously, where you are heading will affect what you take. If you are going to dip a toe in the Arctic Circle, your packing

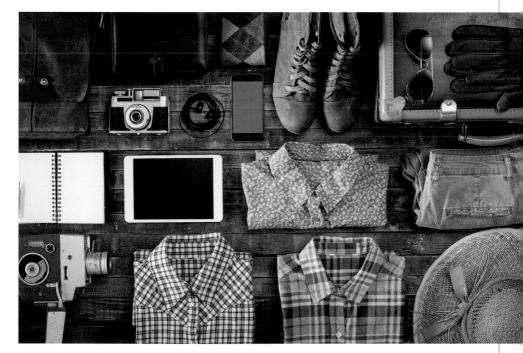

requirements will be different from those of someone preparing to mingle in the markets of Morocco. You don't need to be told that.

Overpacking is a real issue for novice vanners, though. Jumpers and jackets take up loads of space, so finding one good jumper or hoodie that can tolerate the rough and tumble of a laundrette or campsite washing machine is more important than taking the ones that will look great on Instagram. Ditto with a jacket. While the average outdoor jacket is not the most stylish piece of outerwear, a good one will roll up small, stand up to persistent rain and not be too warm if it turns out nice. Unless you are heading to polar bear country or have masses of storage, you will regret packing your parka. More thin layers are better than fewer thick ones.

Footwear

Similarly, keep a tight rein on your footwear. One pair of good shoes that are tough enough for footpaths and smart enough to wear to dinner will be invaluable. Trainers are great for comfort but all that pleather and plastic is a recipe for ripe odours – unbearable in a tight space. Once trainers get wet, baked and sweaty enough times, they will hum, regardless of impeccable foot hygiene. Natural materials are best here.

That said, a pair of sliders, sandals or flip-flops that can be tucked in a corner near the door are a must-have for wandering about the van, site or stopover without the hassle of lacing up every time you head out.

Kitchenalia

If you poke your head around the door of a van being used by first-time vanners, you are likely to see a sea of plastic tat from camping accessory shops. Do the same observation on a seasoned vanner's kitchen cupboard and you'll see a collection of items that look eerily similar to those you might use at home. That's because the vast majority of stuff sold specifically for caravan and motorhome use is novelty junk.

Collapsible kettles, cutlery sets that clip together, mess tins and melamine mugs will all make you feel like you are being punished rather than enjoying yourself, so should really be avoided.

Instead, go for fewer, better-quality items. A good general knife, kept sharp, a bread knife and a handful of regular domestic cutlery are enough to cope with 90 per cent of culinary requirements. A vegetable peeler is a luxury, but a worthwhile addition; a tin opener is a must for nights where anything more challenging than a tin of soup is too much effort; and a small chopping board is crucial. If you are cheffy, get two, so you can chop your meat and veg separately without having to keep rinsing things. A good saucepan and a small frying pan are essential, but make sure they fit in whatever cupboard space you have available. It goes without saying that a top-quality bottle opener should be packed. In fact, it's always worth keeping a spare, just in case.

In terms of prettiness, not much beats enamel plates and mugs. They are tough, too, but the mugs in particular can be a bit of a chore as they get so hot to the touch. Packed carefully, regular porcelain mugs bring a touch of civility to proceedings. The same goes for glassware. Get something compact and don't spend a fortune, then pack them in tea towels to ensure they survive the journey and to minimise clatter as you roll down the road.

Staying connected

As recently as a decade ago, we'd be discussing laptops, modems and all manner of other paraphernalia, but the boundless progress of mobile phone technology means that today you need little more than that to keep your fans apprised of your progress.

Increasingly, campsites, service stations, coffee shops and pretty much everywhere else have Wi-Fi hotspots so you need not rack up huge bills, either. The main thing to be mindful of is the availability of power to keep these little pocket computers fully topped up.

If your van doesn't have them already, consider fitting some USB power sockets, ideally rigged up to your leisure battery. That way, you won't be relying on a mains connection or wobbly cigar lighter 12v charger to stay powered up.

If you really rely on having connectivity on the go, invest in a personal Wi-Fi hotspot with its own SIM card, and possibly an external antenna. Now that roaming charges across Europe have been somewhat normalised, at least across EU countries, this is now a good-value option for those who need to be on the net all the time.

⬇ A laptop and a phone with a suitable data contract are all you need to stay connected when you are on the road.

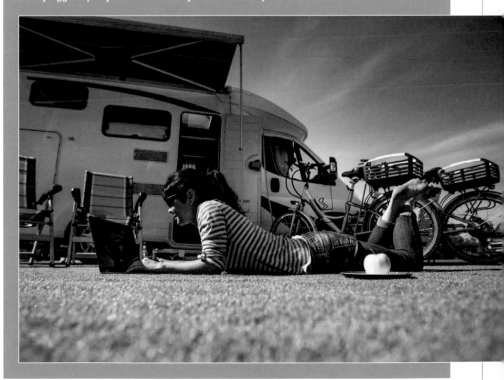

Saving money

Before hitting the road, many people put a lot of effort into saving money, whether by setting some funds aside every month or perhaps committing an amount of their pension to realise their dream.

With that much effort going into saving beforehand, it makes sense that an equal amount goes into budgeting once you are on the road to make that money go as far as it possibly can.

If you are away for a few weeks, it'll be fine to just pitch up your van at sites as you find them. For longer trips or extended stays, however, very low-cost or free overnight spots make a lot of sense. In the UK, membership of one of the two main caravan clubs is a good idea, and if you are travelling with a caravan, essential.

There are differences between the two clubs, but ostensibly, they both offer excellent support for caravan and motorhome owners. Both have a wide network of high-quality sites available at discounted rates for members, and among them are some of the best-located ones in the country. If you want to get lochside in Scotland or among the lakes in Cumbria, you'll get your money's worth in no time at all. Both clubs also offer excellent insurance products, local groups for socialising, rallies, temporary sites and all manner of extra value that may not be immediately apparent.

Perhaps the best benefit of all, though, is the network of secret sites that are only open to club members. As a caravan user, you cannot stop stealthily down a quiet road in the same way as a discreet campervan; you will always need to find a site. Big commercial sites are often filled at peak periods but if you dip into the club's small site network, there is generally a pitch nearby you probably didn't know was there, and at an eye-catching price to boot.

The Caravan and Motorhome Club (formerly the Caravan Club) call their small sites Certificated Locations (CL), while the Camping and Caravanning Club call their ones Certificated Sites (CS). Essentially, they are bound by the same rules – namely that no more than five vans can stay at any one time, and that they all provide a fresh water supply and a place in which to empty waste and toilet tanks. The maximum length of continuous stay is 28 days.

Commercial sites cost upwards of £20 per night, even in the low season, and those costs soon mount up, but typical CL and CS costs can on occasion give you change from £10, depending on what facilities they offer.

Standard facilities are predictably basic, but many go beyond; all-weather pitches, shower blocks, laundry and mains electric hook-ups are often available for a modest extra charge.

The Caravan and Motorhome Club has more than 2,500 of these sites in the UK, while the Camping and Caravanning Club has more than 1,400. If you are long-term touring or full-timing, these small site networks are invaluable for managing your outgoings. Along with the other savings, membership fees for either club – at around £50 – quickly look like good value. For wider travelling, the C&MC's *Touring*

Making money

We've mentioned the rise of the digital nomad already, but if you don't happen to be blessed with programming skills or some other talent that allows you to feather your nest from afar, there are other options.

One very popular choice is to get work as a seasonal campsite warden. Clubs and commercial sites take on people in this manner, allowing them to flexibly staff up for the high season, with a discounted pitch supplied as part of the remuneration. If you don't object to a bit of grass cutting, cleaning and manning reception desks, it is a nice way to spend a summer season while topping up your coffers.

If you have a specific talent and if you are staying in an area for a while, you can stick a note (with permission) in the window of the local tabac or village noticeboard to advertise whatever service you can offer. Gardening, decorating or basic handyman skills are always in demand, and if you are near an expat area, you may find someone with an accent you recognise who would like to have a gossip about what is going on at home while you make yourself useful. Do be mindful, however, that once people think you are essentially on 'holiday', they may think you are helping them out as a favour. Ensure the remuneration is discussed up front, especially if you are working for other van owners or expat locals.

At the traditional end are the more back-breaking tasks such as fruit picking and packing up the harvest at the correct time of year. That sort of work is not as easy to find as it once was, but if you speak the local language well enough then ask the question. If you have sufficient language skills to count and understand a drinks order, then a bit of casual bar work is always an option, and you'll never be short of someone to share a pint with.

In all cases, be mindful of local sensitivities when looking for casual employment opportunities. If there is a local gardener or handyman, they may not take kindly to a hostile takeover of their livelihood from some van-dwelling fly-by-night. If you are in town for a shortish stay and looking for work, stick to labouring and simple stuff to steer clear of any local hostility. That way, your employer can take up the issue with anyone who objects.

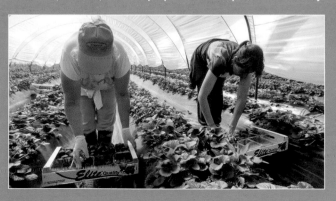

← Labouring tasks like fruit picking are often available seasonally. It's only for the physically fit however!

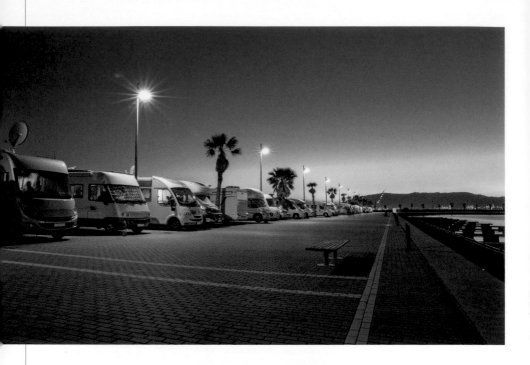

books are essential. They list basically every site you'll find across the countries covered, with up-to-date reviews of facilities, price info and detailed directions which are suitable for larger vehicles. The guides are available to non-members, but they are charged more.

Aside from major club membership, it's also worth looking into camping cards for Europe. The ACSI Camping Card caps site fees in low season on participating sites. Discounts are claimed at 'up to 50%' but 25 per cent is more typical. There are even some UK sites in the guidebook that is supplied with the card, so you know which parks to aim for to get the best deals. With more than 3,300 sites across more than a dozen European countries, it is definitely worth investing in the card if you are spending time on the Continent. It is available from Vicarious Books, who are the UK distributor. Head to

↑ Specialist guide books will point you in the direction of the best stopping places and overnight spots for your van.

www.vicariousbooks.co.uk to get your copy for under £20.

Depending on where you are heading, it is also worth investigating the Camping Key Europe. This has replaced something called the Camping Card Scandinavia, but basically does the same thing. It is accepted as an ID card at sites that require you to keep your ID for the duration of your stay, which is worth the charge alone. The camping key also qualifies users for discounts from sites using the scheme. The majority of those that do are in Sweden, Denmark, Norway and Finland, but if you are heading that way, anything that helps bring costs down is very worthwhile. Find details at www.campingkeyeurope.com.

Free parking

To many, the real freedom of your own accommodation is the ability to stop wherever you please. That is a lovely idea, and to an extent, it is entirely possible. In certain places, and with the right precautions taken.

First things first – if this is your dream, then you really need to drop any ideas of owning a caravan. While there are some places where it is not entirely prohibited to wild camp in a caravan, you will always be more conspicuous and less welcome in trailered accommodation.

In the UK, even with a camper or motorhome, free or wild camping is, frankly, difficult. It is not impossible however. There are excellent resources built by the motorhome community which indicate places where you can enjoy a quiet night or two, but it will always be a little uncertain. That said, councils and local law enforcement have better things to do than go looking for discreetly parked motorhomes.

There are some common sense rules that can help you work out whether your overnight halt is a good idea or not.

Stay well away from buildings, and if at all possible, sneak your van behind a natural barrier such as a hedge or tree line. Private property is to be avoided without permission of the land owner and never drive through a gate or barrier which is open to find a stop. It might be closed when you come back.

Bear in mind that you should avoid alcohol if parking without permission. If you get moved on, you need to be fit to drive.

For information on well-researched UK stops, check out the Brit Stops website which is an excellent resource and should

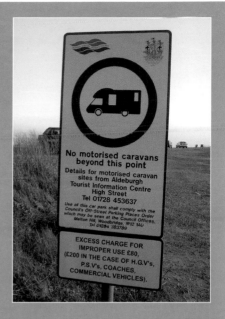

ensure you never get caught out. *Practical Motorhome* magazine also maintains a small list of free (or very low cost) Nightstops. Both should be in your internet bookmarks.

Away from the UK, wild camping is a very different prospect. The Scandinavian countries all allow visitors the right to explore common land. Be considerate, leave things as you find them and you can stay where you please.

Across pretty much everywhere else in Europe, there are affordable overnight stop networks which are well documented on the Park4Night website amongst others. If you want to keep it analogue, Vicarious Books has country-specific guides to all the places you are likely to patronise.

http://www.britstops.com
https://practicalmotorhome.com/nightstops
https://park4night.com
https://www.vicarious-shop.com

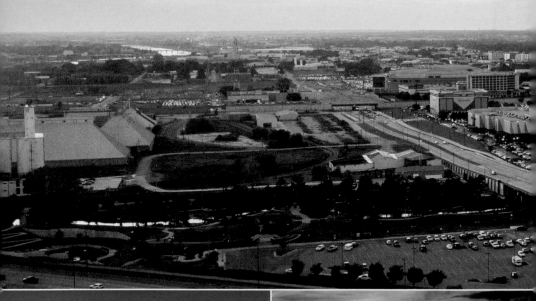

Van Life Inspiration

Route 66,
The USA

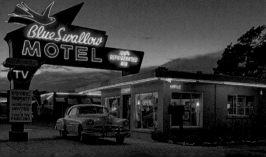

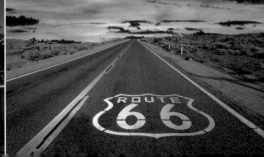

The Mother Road, as Route 66 is also known, was one of the original US highways but its full extent existed for only 59 years. Tracing the original 2,500-mile route from Chicago to Los Angeles is now impossible. But there is enough of it left, enough that is preserved and enough folk hungry to find it, to keep it as the world's favourite bucket list highway.

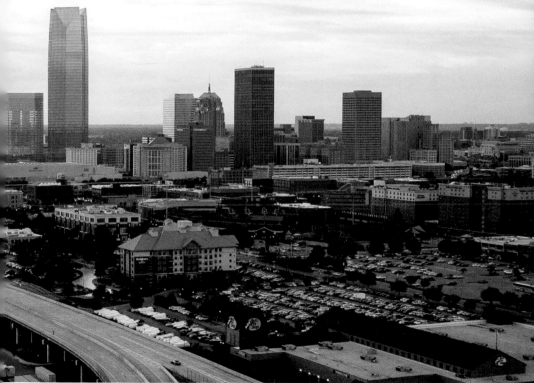

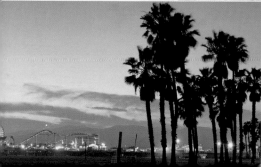

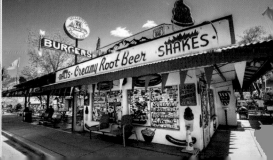

Index